# Not Your Mother's Book...
## On SEX

Created and Edited by
Dahlynn McKowen,
Ken McKowen and Pamela Frost

D1715719

Published by
Publishing Syndicate LLC

PO Box 607
Orangevale California 95662
www.PublishingSyndicate.com

# Not Your Mother's Book . . .

## On SEX

Copyright 2015 by Publishing Syndicate LLC

*We would like to thank the many individuals
who granted us permission to print their stories.
See the complete listing beginning on page 322.*

Edited by Dahlynn McKowen,
Ken McKowen and Pamela Frost
Cover and Book Design by Publishing Syndicate
Cover photo: alphaspirit/Shutterstock.com
Copyeditor: Dahlynn McKowen
Proofreader: Pat Nelson

Published by
**Publishing Syndicate** LLC
PO Box 607
Orangevale California 95662

www.PublishingSyndicate.com
www.Facebook.com/PublishingSyndicate
Twitter: @PublishingSynd

Print Edition ISBN: 978-1-938778-42-1
EPUB Digital Edition ISBN: 978-1-938778-44-5
MOBI Digital Edition ISBN 978-938778-43-8
Library of Congress Control Number
2014911844

Printed in Canada.

This book is a collaborative effort. Writers from all over the world submitted their work for consideration, with 69 stories making the final cut.

Publishing Syndicate strongly encourages you to submit your story for one of its many upcoming anthologies.

For information on how to submit your story, go to www.PublishingSyndicate.com.

# CONTENTS

## 4  What's the Speed Limit of Sex?

## 5  What's the Expiration Date of Sex?

## 6  Sex and the Digital Age

## 7  Afraid to Ask . . .

## 12  Shhh, Let It Happen . . .

# Introduction

*Those who are easily shocked should be shocked more often.*

-- Mae West

## SEX! SEX! SEX and MORE SEX!

That's what I'm talking about.

It's said that food, clothing and shelter are the necessities of life. Really? Without sex, we wouldn't even be here. It's a biological fact. The sex drive is strong for a reason—the species must continue at all costs.

When it comes to life's necessities, for me, sex is number one, followed closely by a sense of humor. In my humble opinion, life without sex and laughter would not be worth living. And chocolate. Where's my chocolate? But I digress.

So I ask you, what would be better than a book that takes a peek under the covers and behind closed doors to shine a light on the comical antics of those lovable humans and their sexual encounters? Nothing would be better. I mean, you can't be having sex *all* the time. So fill that time between orgasms with laughter and a good book—this book.

Yes, this book! Sex and laughter conveniently packaged together for your stimulating pleasure. In the pages that follow, you will not find graphic blow-by-blow descriptions of sexual acts. Well, maybe that one story . . . but no, not really. You *will* giggle at the mishaps of sex, like punctured waterbeds, the truth behind the combination of sex and whipped cream, and, of course, the ever-popular combination of cars and sex.

If you pee your pants laughing when reading *Vaginaplasty*, you might need one. If you're prone to this problem, you'll want to take precautions before reading *Do You Vajazzle?* You've been warned. And you will find stories of young lust that will warm the cockles of your heart. Caution: If your cockles become too warm, rub with dry ice.

You will also find a new look at old fairy tales, such as Cinderella explaining how she really found her Prince Charming, codpiece and all. And who could forget shopping? That's another necessity of life, especially when shopping for vibrating plastic male parts or the perfectly sexy outfit to wear—or peel off.

This book spans the ages from "the talk" to cougars. We even offer advice, with tongue firmly planted in check (or somewhere else) in the chapter, "Kick Him to the Curb." Then, in the interest of equality, men have their say in their very own chapter.

So read on. I invite you to live vicariously through these stories, get aroused and dream about your own fantasies. And if this book doesn't make you laugh, you might want to see a doctor about that stick up your ass.

~~ Pamela Frost

*The 1960s are gone, dope will never be as cheap,*
*sex never as free, and the rock and roll never as great.*
~~ Abbie Hoffman

CHAPTER ONE

# Costumes and Props Required

And don't forget the batteries!

# How to Buy a Plastic Penis

by
Pamela Frost

There are times in a woman's life when a plastic penis is far more satisfying than the flesh-and-blood role model. Post-divorce is one of those times. After a while, I found my hands were not getting me to where I needed to be. And I soon grew bored with vegetables. The mere act of standing in the grocery store staring at a vegetable—trying to figure out if it's the right size and the right texture—felt weird. I wondered if there really were people in the world who could read minds. I just didn't like taking those kinds of chances in public.

So I asked my friend one night while she had a mouth full of wine, "How would one go about buying a plastic penis?" Note to self . . . apparently chardonnay burns when it comes through your nose. When her coughing subsided, she strained to say, "Adam and Eve dot com."

I ran to the computer as soon as I got home.

The banner on the website read, "Top 5 Most Orgasmic Ideas for Summer Fun!" I felt my heart rate increase. And I learned that if I were to sign up right then and there, I could save $10 instantly.

Another note to self: delete browser history. I didn't know how I'd explain this to my son.

I scrolled down the page—fake man parts, fake lady parts, lingerie and so much more. The first thing that caught my eye was something called "Clone-a-Willy." *What in the world? There's something I'll probably never see on Pinterest*, I said to myself. I stand corrected. I *did* find it on Pinterest.

Getting back to Adam and Eve, I clicked the link for Clone-a-Willy. It was a kit to make your own vibrator. I am a do-it-yourselfer, so this idea appealed to me. However, it wasn't going to work for me because the kit required a male to slip his erection into the warm molding liquid. I didn't have access to an erection—he got custody of that in the divorce.

I navigated to the vibrator section. There were seven different categories of vibrators. I was feeling a little over-whelmed when I spotted a tab that read, "For beginners." *How considerate of them to help us newbies.*

Again, too many categories. The first choice was "rabbit vibrators." *Why a rabbit? Oh, I see. Little bunny ears caress the clitoris.* As I scrolled down the page, a staggering array of shapes came alive before my eyes. It took me a minute or so to figure out what might go where. *All three at once?* My imagination ran wild. There were 19 different rabbits to choose from. *This is the beginners' page?!*

Next, I chose the dildo tab. *Now that's what I need . . . something that actually looks like a penis.* Only there were 38 different kinds and many of them didn't look like any dicks I had ever seen. *They come that big in real life? Never in mine. What have I been missing?*

My loins began to stir just looking at all the plastic penises—two pages' worth. This was harder than picking out a zucchini. I settled on a nice mid-sized, mid-priced model that looked like a penis and not some appendage from an outer-space alien. And it was only $24.95.

I clicked, and another box popped up, sharing info on other things I very well could need to go with my plastic penis. *They really have thought of everything on this site.*

The first suggestion was lube. *That makes sense.* Toy cleaner. *Oh yes, that's a must. At least I'll know where this penis has been, but still, cleaner is better.*

Then something called "Make Me Cum" popped up onto the screen. *No, wait, I don't want that.* I wanted to prolong my fun. *Pass.* And finally, mini nipple suckers, recommended for solo masturbation. *Check.* I added those to my cart. That's when I was told I would receive a free mystery gift toy or CD. *Hooray!* But wait, there's more! I was offered a five-piece ultimate orgasm kit. *Yes, that's what I'm talkin' about.*

It was time to check out. That's when I hesitated, right before I clicked the "Pay Now" button. I felt like such a pervert. I reasoned that if I was a pervert for ordering a plastic penis by mail, at least I wasn't alone. From the looks of the website, this company had sold more than a few plastic man-replacement tools.

I couldn't help myself. Before I placed my order, I opened another browser tab and Googled "sex toy sales." I learned that sex toys are a $15-billion-a-year industry. I also found an article explaining sex toy sales per capita, which included a list of the 10 states that bought the most. Wyoming was number one! *Guess it gets pretty lonely out there in the middle of nowhere.* Alaska was number two. *For the same reason, I suppose.* Californians and New Yorkers didn't even make the top 10. *Guess they're too busy enjoying the real thing, and I'm not talking about Coca-Cola.*

That's when one last thought crossed my mind: *If I place this order, I could catapult Ohio into the top 10!* A girl's gotta try.

*Click.* Order submitted.

Let's hear it for Ohio!

# This Calls for a Thong

by
Cynthia Ballard Borris

"So, how was your anniversary?" I asked my friend as I dipped a tortilla chip into the bowl of salsa. "I can't believe you two have hit silver.

"Twenty-five years, same guy." Barb lifted her glass and drew a gentle sip of her tequila. "Same old, same old."

"I heard you went to Vegas to celebrate. How romantic," I said. Looking at my empty ring finger, I wondered, *One life, one man. Imagine building memories together cuddled in the same arms every night. Hmm? Nah, I love my life. Adventuresome, spontaneous and unpredictable. I can buy my own ring.*

"I fell asleep," Barb said. She slumped against the back of the booth.

"But that was after the candles and Champagne, right?"

A negative nod from Barb confirmed the anniversary had gone south. She gazed at a couple at the bar who were lost in a kiss.

"You mean not even a little 'wham-bam'—you know— 'thank-you-ma'am'?" I was pushing the envelope of friendship.

"We have that every night." She broke a chip in half. It dropped into the salsa and sank.

I stared at the woman across from me and gulped. "Every night?"

"Pretty routine. Lights out, covers back, in-and-out stuff."

"Best bud, you owe this guy." Grabbing her arm, I continued. "Come on. We're going to Macy's lingerie department." I dropped a $20 onto the table then added, "And boy, does he owe you."

Warm under the influence of tequila, we trekked to the underwear department on Macy's third floor. Felina, Oscar de la Renta, Calvin Klein taunted and teased. French cut, high cut, no cut whispered in sensual vibes, "Oh baby, oh baby, oh baby."

I headed for the Cosabella section. I loved the cut, the sensual colors and the celebration of sexuality.

"What's that?" I asked Barb, wryly studying the white cotton briefs with blue flowers she had in her hands. "Are you planning to go skydiving?"

A perplexed look clouded her face, canceling out her tequila high.

I took the panties from her and stretched them seam to seam, peeking around the three-layer absorbent panel. "You could use this as a parachute."

"But they're buy two, get one free," she countered and

started to fill her arms with the cotton bounty.

It was worse than I had anticipated. As I took her by the hand, those panties, which had more coverage than an insurance policy, tumbled onto the ground.

"This calls for a thong." I thumbed through the racks of delicate wisps of strings and tapped my finger on the silver metal bar. "What size? Medium?"

"I couldn't wear one of these," Barb said. She dangled the strip of material on her index finger and whispered, "Isn't it uncomfortable?"

"Of course it's uncomfortable." I snagged three items and held them up to the light for a better look. "But then, you're not supposed to be in them long." I nudged her with my elbow and smiled. "That's the point."

"Take a look at this one," I said, showing my friend a pair of shimmering blue panties, dotted with rhinestones. The floss of a thong wore a price tag of $25.

"You mean someone would really wear these?" Barb asked, now dropping to a bare hush.

We moved from display to display, sifting through everything from endowed bras to sheer-to-the-nipple. Arms overloaded with elegant bras and skimpy panties, we paraded into the dressing room. I stripped down to the bare necessities and slid the filmy intimates off hangers. Adorned in my sexuality, I posed forward and backward and pursed my lips to the mirrors. I waved to the hidden-camera operator.

"Oh, my God," I heard Barb say. Hangers rattled inside her dressing room, which was next to mine.

I pulled the pleated curtain aside and there stood Barb

in a feathery green outfit. I affirmed her comment. "Oh, my God," I said, covering my mouth to inhale a snicker. "Maybe neon green isn't your color." I choked on the words. "And feathers!"

A defeated gaze reflected in the mirror as she sighed. "Maybe I should just go home and soak in a hot bath."

"Not unless he's in it with you," I said, noting to look for bubble bath and floating candles.

"This is so not me," she said, still looking at her reflection. A plucked feather drifted to the carpet. "It's hopeless."

"Try again." I closed the curtain and waited for the next floorshow.

"Maybe it'd be easier to just roll over and go to sleep," Barb offered from the other side.

"No way. This is serious business. You're in trouble, girlfriend—in the bedroom department!" I shouted back, "Come on. Bare that booty!"

"OK, here I come." She parted the drape.

Tight buns . . . orange thong . . . *what?!* There was a cartoon character on the front of her . . . *what?!* I pushed the little nose on the fuzzy bear that was inches below her belly button, and it played a sorrowful rendition of *Tonight's the Night.*

I shoved Barb back into the cubicle and said, "Next?!"

While she continued trying on outfits, I changed back into my clothes.

"Hmm? Yeah," I heard from the other side of the curtain. Barb came out wearing a red, easy-on-the-eye lace bra and matching panties.

"Wait." I hustled back to the racks of seduction-in-wait and looked for the missing accessory. I searched the delicate laces then there it was. It was perfect.

"Here." I tossed the item into her dressing stall.

"Is this a . . . ?"

"Yes. It's a snug-to-fit, guaranteed-to-please, garter belt." I leaned against the wall, arms crossed over chest, satisfied with my mission. *Score one for best buds.*

Barb left the store with a small package of lust under her arm. I bought something, too, because that's what friends do.

I hugged Barb goodbye and hopped into my Toyota.

The next morning, midway between my cinnamon scone and French roast, the phone rang. I knew who it was.

"He loved it!" she said. Her excitement rang rich with freshness. "He can't thank you enough." I sensed a purr.

Leaning back in my chair, wrapped warm in familiarity, I said, "Want to go out again next week? I know this great toy store that specializes in . . ."

# The Hired Man

by
### Rae Ellen Lee

"I have a confession to make," my 60-year-old husband, Tom, said. Since our life together had featured a lot of heavy-weather sailing, there wasn't much he could say to shock me.

"Let's hear it," I said, sitting down on the bed in our tiny Caribbean cottage, Villa Debris.

He reached into the closet we shared and brought out my goddess dress. "I've been wearing this, off and on."

"Get your own dress. You're too big. I don't want you wrecking the seams."

A friend had helped me pick out the dress on a trip to St. Croix. It was two separate sleeveless dresses designed to be worn one over the other. I loved the pattern of vertical stripes of lime, teal, hibiscus red and mango on a background of purple shadows. The scoop-neck dress was a filmy rayon concoction that draped over my curves all the way down to my ankles. The slits up both sides to mid-thigh were such a tease that even I felt sexy wearing it.

"Boy, are you lucky," I said, examining the dress. "The seams are still OK."

I got up and walked over to the wicker baskets where I stored my underwear, hearing my flip-flops slapping the tile floor as I made my way. Underneath one of the cats curled up asleep in the basket, I found what I was looking for.

"Here," I said, handing Tom a black half-slip. "You can wear this. It's too long for me to wear with any of my dresses."

"You sure?"

I shrugged. "Yeah, I'm sure." I thought this was probably just a new compulsion of his, one of many obsessions that had come and gone, never to be mentioned again. Over the 10 years we'd been married, there had been the winter of studying for the ham radio instead of finding work; the sled-dog team; acquiring goats to train as pack animals; preparing to ski the Haute Route in Europe; and grinding his own flour. Just to name a few.

Next, Tom showed me his new panties for men, called Manties . . . and a yellow thong like the bushmen wear.

"Oh, a penie guard," I said.

He seemed delighted with his new apparel. "It's getting late," he said. "The new sex toys can wait."

The next day I pondered Tom's latest interest. Did he anticipate my question, "What's in this for me?" Is that why he ordered the sex toys? And what kind of paraphernalia could he be talking about? I had never been into kinky stuff, which reminded me of a funny saying: "Kinky is using a feather; perverted is using the whole chicken." I hoped the sex toys were more feathers than chicken.

I smiled as I puttered around the place, glancing every now and then at the view of the Caribbean out the wall of windows. Paradise had its pitfalls—like dust and bugs and mold—and the windows got dirty so quickly. I wanted to wash them. I really did. But instead, I turned my attention to my desk. When I needed staples for my tiny stapler, I descended the exterior wooden steps to the office/guest room. As soon as I slid open the glass door and entered the musty room, there they were . . . termite tunnels running all over the bookshelves. I grabbed an armload of books and fled the scene.

When I called Tom at work, he said, "I didn't notice any termite tunnels, and I've been down there every morning and night on my computer. I can hardly believe it."

"What have you been doing down there?"

There was no answer at the other end of the phone.

We had a lively evening as Tom entertained me with show and tell. First, he introduced me to the selection of sex toys he had purchased. One of them, "The Hired Man," was made of high-tech silicone. He presented it to me with both hands, as if it were on a silver platter.

"Oh, yeah!" I said. "This thing has some heft to it." It was neither a feather nor a chicken, but it was a sight to behold.

The saying, "Oh, yeah!" always made us laugh. We'd watched exactly one porno movie during our 10-year marriage. The woman in the movie kept saying, "Oh, yeah!" over and over, even though she did not appear to be enjoying what she was doing. It's hard to get some images out of your head.

"You can imagine how long it took to research these things on the Internet using dial-up," Tom confided in earnest, as if sharing a shopping tip. "It can take a long time for a dildo to load, depending on its size."

We laughed like crazy people. The way sound carried on the moist air near the ocean, the neighbor bachelors must have wondered about us. When I recovered, I asked, "What else you got there?"

Tom's face was a little red as he handed me a gelatinous pink thing, about 3 inches long and a couple of inches in diameter. When I turned it on end, I saw that the center of the lewd squishy deal was open all the way through.

"It's called 'The Pocket Rocket,' " he said. "It's guaranteed to send a guy right into orbit."

One night later in the week, while I was sitting on the bed reading, Tom came upstairs from his office and reached for his small duffel bag full of sex toys.

"I became aroused while researching those Seal A Meal devices," he said, matter-of-factly, as he headed back downstairs with the duffel bag.

This small home appliance was a popular item in the islands. When you used one to seal up things like shoes or books or articles of clothing, they wouldn't get moldy. We'd talked about getting one, and I guess tonight was the night. Later, when he came back upstairs and hung the duffel bag on the wall, he told me he'd ordered a Seal A Meal device off eBay. I didn't ask him any other questions, even though I wondered if he'd still keep our appointment for sex tomorrow.

In the morning, he was up for sex as scheduled. But, frankly, I wasn't that interested. Over the next couple of years, I would learn that love at the soul level has nothing to do with gender. But at the time, I did the best I could, which I felt was admirable. With a little help from The Hired Man, we were under the sheet, all lubed up, going at it with limited success. Off and on, I said, "Oh, yeah!" But really, I was thinking about washing the windows in the living room.

All of a sudden, our black cat pounced on us from the rafters. Tom leaped up, the cat flew into the air and I started cussing. Talk about coitus interruptus. And as the particles of dust, mold and cat hair settled, my first thought was, *Well, all right, then. I guess I can go wash those windows.*

Later that night, as we drifted off to sleep, smiling, I thought, *I should just relax about Tom's exploration of all things sexual.* This could be an exciting new chapter in our lives. In fact, I felt certain I was falling in love with The Hired Man. If only he did windows.

# Hair Today

by
Elaine Person

Lance and I had been dating for a few months when I decided it was time to invite him to my place.

I was not the neatest housekeeper, so this was a test. If Lance could handle my sloppiness and quirky personality, we could be a match. If he was flexible, we might progress to a long-term status. And maybe then—just then—I could bring this relationship to the next level. I had heard that sloppy housekeepers were good in bed—he had told me he was a lousy housekeeper, too.

I phoned him early one morning. "Lance, will you help me color my hair tonight? Yes? Then meet me at my place at 6:30 P.M." I gave him my address.

Placing the receiver in its cradle, I realized my back was still sore from a recent car accident. Before I left for work that morning, I used my electric vibrator to release the pain. The vibrator served many purposes, and I used it on many different body parts, whether they were sore or not. It was constructed with a separate, hand-held body and a variety of interchangeable heads: small, rounded and rubbery for frontal fun; flat, like a small sander, for larger areas; plastic, concentric circles with a bull's-eye for back massages; and a metal disc stamped with the word *Heat* for use everywhere.

I sailed through my workday, and Lance was on time. He met me on my front porch as I arrived home from work. We kissed hello on the welcome mat then I unlocked the door. We walked into my apartment together, and I flipped on the light switch. But the living room light didn't come on.

"Wait here," I said and headed to the bedroom. I tried the switch in there—no light came on. I hit the TV remote, to no avail. I tried a few more switches then realized what had happened. I returned to my patient visitor.

"I forgot to pay the electric bill," I admitted. "Their business office is closed until tomorrow morning."

"I guess we shouldn't color your hair in the dark, right? Let's get something to eat in a place that has electricity."

*He handled this well*, I thought. Off we went to Perkins Restaurant.

"Nice to see you again," the server said to Lance and me. I made a face at her, indicating that she had never seen Lance before. *Please don't confuse him with the man I was in here with the other day*, I hoped my pleading look said to her. I was still testing the dating waters with several men simultaneously to see which one rose to the top.

"Good to see you, too," I responded, changing the subject quickly by asking her about the specials.

After Lance and I ate dinner and chatted for a while, he drove me home. We kissed goodbye outside my door.

"Will you please return tomorrow to complete our task?" I said, winking.

"Of course," Lance said, "I can't wait to get my hands on your hair."

After a dark night's sleep and a no-coffee, uncooked breakfast, I called the electric company, paid the delinquent bill over the phone and left for work.

When I returned home, I met Lance at my door again. We entered. I flipped the switch, and the light came on. Then I heard it—a noise coming from the bedroom. I froze. *Who's in there? Thieves? The maintenance crew? Was I ever going to be alone with Lance in my own home?*

Lance heard it, too. Together, we tiptoed toward my bedroom. The buzzing got louder. Following the sound to the floor under my bed, I realized that my vibrator had come on when the power came back on. The head of it was so hot that the metal stem had become disfigured, rotating in a circle like a staggering drunk instead of standing upright. And the heat had burned an indentation in the carpet. I switched the instrument off.

"I ruined the apartment's carpet. I'll have to pay to replace it. And I destroyed my vibrator. I guess I left it turned on," I said to my date while holding up the toy/massage therapist. He learned about me in those four sentences.

Lance laughed. "Don't worry about it. Come on. Let's color your hair."

The next day, I took the vibrator to a small-appliance

repair shop. The owner's wife said, "I can't fix it, but I'll have my husband look at it." Two weeks later, I went to pick it up. I still had not heard from Lance. The woman said, "It can't be fixed. It's worn-out. What did you do to it?"

I didn't answer. I looked at the wilted appliance.

Even my vibrator jilted me.

# My Visit to the Pleasure Chest

by
Marion Hussey

"You want to go *where?!*" I asked my pal Cindy.

"I think we should pay a visit to the Pleasure Chest." She made the suggestion as if it was a simple trip to the grocery store.

I had heard about the Pleasure Chest in West Hollywood for years, knowing it was the supermarket of sex toys. I always wondered what kind of bounty waited inside the walls of this establishment, but I was afraid to go by myself.

"Game on," I agreed. The following weekend, the two of us trekked into the sordid side of West Hollywood to explore this new terrain.

The first rack inside the door featured risqué greeting cards. Hunky boy's birthday greetings, transvestite tribulations and everything in between paid homage to various flights of fancy in the sexual arena. I had expected to see call girls, gigolos and other colorful characters, but the patrons seemed pretty tame. Many couples walked down the aisles as if they were shopping at Walmart.

We soon grew bored with the cards and decided to venture deeper into the store. On the right were a variety of lubricants and gels and other wet things designed to enhance penetration and massage.

*Now we are getting somewhere,* I said to myself, fondling an amber-colored bottle shaped like a phallus. I dropped a bottle of cinnamon stick into my basket and wandered across the aisle toward the rubber instruments.

Cindy beat me to the rack, holding up a double-headed dildo as if it was a victory sword. "On guard!" Then she started fencing with it as we both gazed at its tremendous girth.

I picked up a 4-pound rubber cock. "Who could take this in?"

"Maybe it's for a donkey," replied Cindy, pretending to insert it into her mouth.

Dildos in a variety of colors stood at attention. There were black ones, beige ones and several pink dildos in a variety of shapes. And there were many in colors I'm sure never occur in nature. Some had ridges, some required batteries and some were a complete mystery. *Hopefully those come with instruction manuals.*

Further into the heart of the store, I came across another rubber section, entitled "Pep Boys." I knew it wasn't a tire store! One apparatus looked like some sort of mask with a hose attached. I was too embarrassed to ask the salesperson what it was for, preferring to use my imagination and pretend that it was a sexual device for snorkelers.

In the fashion aisle, there were feather boas, festive masks and other delights that put me right on Bourbon Street during Mardi Gras. Next to the feathers were a variety of leather contraptions and restraints, reminding me of books by Henry Miller, Anaïs Nin and Charles Bukowski.

I knew my knowledge of S&M was rather rudimentary—compared with that of some of my more experienced friends—so these instruments put a fresh spin on what I already knew. I had heard about S&M bars where members were allowed to participate or simply sit around and see what happens. *Do they bring these toys? Maybe you can just rent them?* Perhaps I should've brought these friends to the Pleasure Chest with us so they could explain the nuances of these devices.

Since I was newly single, I decided to invest in some items to expand my appeal. Hey, being single is all about marketing, and I knew I had to extend my brand. I bought a few dildos in various sizes and a vibrator, too. They were even on sale!

And that was my first visit to the Pleasure Chest, but certainly not my last. New lovers have their preferences, and, of course, that warrants another shopping trip to Santa Monica Boulevard, where rubber rules and feathers fly.

# Searching for Mr. Right . . . Size

by
Stephen Vanek

Size doesn't matter. It's how you use it that matters. Right?

That's the polite, I-love-you-just-the-way-you-are angle girls play with guys. I know that. I'm a guy.

But times change. Face-to-face, I think females probably maintain their polite façade. But more and more, the media is abuzz with talk that is quite contrary. Size *does* matter.

With that in mind and a desire to buy Ginger, my girl-friend, a naughty surprise, I decided to look for a big—I mean *really* big—dildo at a nearby adult toy store.

My size is just fine. At least that's what Ginger assures me, and we fit together nicely. Since the two of us enjoyed experimenting sexually, and bigger was supposed to be better, I went into the store looking for BIG. After wavering on a few dildos that met my specs, I made the decision to buy the "Chad Hunt 12-inch Super Cock."

Yes—12 inches long and as thick as a 10-ounce water bottle. The dildo was flesh colored, rubbery soft, but firm. This erection wasn't going away. And it wasn't cheap either at 80 bucks. Carrying it out of the store, I realized how heavy the thing was. I laughed to myself, thinking, *If it's too big, she can always use it as a hand weight.*

When I arrived at Ginger's place and removed her gift from the bag, her eyes widened. Although she didn't say it, I'm sure she was thinking, "Are you kidding me?" It really was huge. Instead, she smiled, kissed and hugged me, as if I'd invited an intelligent guest to dinner. Ginger's like that.

Still hugging me, Ginger turned to look at it. "That's really big," she said, smirking. "Are guys' cocks really that big?"

No, she hadn't watched a lot of porn. But I had. And to be honest, I'd never seen a guy with a cock as big as this one. Well, maybe once or twice.

"I don't think so," I replied. "I mean, there are a few. Maybe. I guess."

Why was I stammering?

We both gawked at how well-designed it was, with its light flesh color (I'm darker skinned) and how it thrust straight up (I have a distinct left curve). And it swayed slightly after being suctioned to her nightstand (I bob up and down when I stand).

I remember having an unexpected sense that this dildo could be my replacement. I wasn't worried—not at all—but it's a little unnerving staring at a monstrous replica of a penis with the woman you adore, the woman you've fallen head over heels for, the woman you think about doing almost every minute of the day. OK, that's an exaggeration. Kind of.

"I'm going to name him 'Clive,'" Ginger said, running her fingertip over the faux urethra opening. At her touch, Clive swayed on the nightstand.

I might have grimaced, but at least I didn't say what I was thinking, *Isn't it too early in our relationship to give a dildo a name?* What is the rule on when it's appropriate to name a dildo? Could it be I was feeling pangs of jealousy?

Ginger looked at me, a twinkle in her eye, apparently sizing up my confidence. She blurted, "You know, if I use Clive, he's going to stretch me out, and I might not feel you anymore."

I sighed, feeling demoralized. Clive? The dildo was now a "he?" It was a damned rubber cock!

"Are you serious?" I replied, helplessly. I'd never considered the elasticity of her vagina to a particular cock. "Maybe I should take it back?"

But Ginger shook her head and dug in. "You can't return cocks, darling. I think we're stuck with Clive."

I sighed again, a little shrunken at her amusement.

"He's huge," she said, with a burst of you-can't-be-serious laughter. "Can we try him now?"

And so, we did. But Clive, in fact, was too big.

*Oh, darn.*

So what do you do with an $80 dildo named Clive? Mount him as a memento of a sexual escapade gone terribly wrong? Nope. Clive's final resting place ended up being in a box that was shoved into the nether regions of Ginger's closet, far behind clothes she'll probably never wear again.

The moral of the story? Size does matter—the right size.

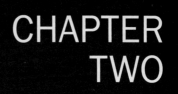
# Best Laid
# Plans . . .

. . . or how *not* to get laid!

# Hard Knocks

by
Marilyn Underwood

Many years ago, my older brother—a confirmed bachelor—surprised us all by getting married. The ceremony was performed in another state, and since no one in my family attended, my mother planned a party a few weeks later to welcome the bride.

I'm from a large family, and my parents' house overflowed with spouses and kids. Thus, my husband and I opted to stay overnight at a hotel. The town was small and our choices were limited. One option was the motel out by the highway. The price was right, but the place was dark, damp and dirty, so we chose the "ritzy" hotel on the town square.

Hotel St. Charles occupied a historic four-story red brick building across the square from the town's 200-year-old Catholic church. With its gleaming white trim and wrought-iron railings, the hotel was the epitome of elegance. The most expensive restaurant in town was located on the main floor, and the hotel had a stellar reputation throughout the region. Being newlyweds ourselves, we were excited to have an excuse to stay in such a fancy place.

The party honoring my brother and his new wife was fun, but by 8 P.M., we'd had enough of the family and were ready for some time alone. When I'd made the reservation, the clerk told me that the hotel's reception desk closed at 10 P.M., and that we needed to arrive before then. By the time we'd said our goodbyes, stopped at the store for a bottle of wine and drove to the hotel, it was nearly 10. The desk clerk was still there and checked us in. Once in our room, we realized that even though it was small, the antique bed and crystal chandelier gave it an air of elegance and romance.

My husband went to look for ice. I took a shower and donned my new negligee.

"They really do close this place down at 10," he said when I emerged from the bathroom. "The reception desk is locked up and there's a sign that says they'll return at 6 A.M., and for emergencies, call 911. I think we have the place to ourselves."

It was shaping up to be quite the romantic weekend. We sipped our wine for a bit, and while my husband showered, I watched a few minutes of *Saturday Night Live*.

Freshly shaved and smelling great, my husband topped off our wine and flipped off the lights and the TV.

"To us!" We clinked our glasses, sipped and . . .

*THUD!*

The sound came from the wall behind our headboard, the wall we shared with the adjacent room.

"I guess we don't have the place to ourselves," whispered my husband.

*THUD!*

"Nope. Not unless it's a ghost," I whispered back.

Then the moans began . . . moans that might have been mistaken for a ghost if not for the liberal sprinkling of phrases like, "Oh, yes," "Oh, God," and "Give me more!"

There's nothing that kills the romantic mood like the knowledge that if you can hear them, they certainly can hear you.

The moaning and groaning and thudding against the wall went on for some time. We whispered about how embarrassed that couple would be if they knew how well they could be heard. It was funny until the neighbors became so raucous that the pictures on the walls rattled and the crystals on the chandelier chattered. We put pillows over our ears, but that didn't block out the sound effects from next door. Finally, the clamor settled into a quiet murmur.

Our romantic evening had been spoiled, but at least the bed was comfortable. Just as I started to drift off, the noises began again.

"You've got to be kidding me," whispered my husband.

"They must have some serious stamina," I whispered back.

The thumping and moaning progressed to the expected conclusion.

The silence was welcome, but it didn't last long.

This time the man was the most vocal participant. I was just about to put the pillow back over my ears when I heard,

"Wait. Stop. Let's do that one again."

The thudding stopped.

The moaning stopped.

Conversation started.

Man's voice.

Woman's voice.

Another man's voice?

"There must be two couples in there," I said quietly.

"I only hear one woman," said my husband.

"But there are definitely two men."

We had just moved from the realm of embarrassing to kinky.

In the quiet, a man said, "Great. Let's get started again."

"Hang on," said the woman. "I gotta go pee."

A door closed, and the men began to talk. Except now, there were three distinct male voices.

And that took us from kinky to holy-crap-twisted.

"This is way too weird," said my husband.

"What do you want to do?" I asked.

"There's not much we can do. We can't change rooms, and this doesn't qualify for a 911 call. We'll have to sleep on the floor if we go to your parents' house. Surely they can't keep it up all night."

"Surely" was wrong.

My husband started snoring around three, but the cater-wauling kept me awake for at least another hour.

The next morning, our neighbors were quiet. Perhaps it had all been some horrible perverted nightmare?

"I think they were filming a skin flick next door," said

my husband when he awoke.

"No way. This isn't LA or Vegas or wherever they make porn. This is small-town Podunk Midwest. They don't do stuff like that here."

"Whatever you say. Let's go find some caffeine."

Fortunately, the restaurant had lots of strong, hot coffee. After a couple of quarts, we felt almost human. While my husband paid the bill, I wandered into the lobby. A man and a woman with two large black trunks stood at the reception desk.

"Did you have a nice night?" asked the perky clerk.

"Sure," said the man.

"That's great! So we'll see you again next Saturday?"

"You bet," he said as he hefted a trunk marked "lights."

By that time, my husband had joined me in the lobby. "Our neighbors?" he asked me.

I shrugged, and we headed upstairs. Just as we reached our floor, two men carrying more trunks came out of the room next to ours. We stepped aside to let them pass. The trunks were labeled "camera" and "props."

Apparently, small-town Podunk Midwest is exactly where they make porn. Every Saturday night.

*The hotel's name has been changed to protect the not-so-innocent.

# But It's My Birthday

by
Georgia Mellie Justad

"It's my birthday!" declared my husband excitedly—again. This three-word phrase soon became a broken record that played for hundreds of miles from southern Florida to northern Georgia, placing me in my own personal hellish version of the movie *Groundhog Day*.

Yeah, it was Hubby's birthday all right, but what those words really meant in the mind of my husband of 20 years was, "I want sex. Now. And lots of it."

For the record, "It's Wednesday" or "It's Friday"—the two days Hubby worked from home—and "Pass the ketchup," translate into the same message. However, "birthday sex," as every woman knows, implies that the men in their lives are entitled to something extra, like a rum floater atop a pina colada. Or, in my case, Russian Kazakh dancing on a tabletop, clad in a Cool Whip cape. Luckily, birthday sex comes only once a year.

Now don't think I'm a prude or anything. I perform my wifely duties on a regular basis, but with our son home for summer break, I had to be creative with time management. Naturally, Hubby—being a man who thinks sex should be as frequent as the mail—will invariably yank me into the storage shed or garage at a moment's notice to steal a little afternoon delight. Speaking for hot-flashing, mood-swinging menopausal women everywhere, let's just say the postman never rings twice at our house.

My baby, a 6-foot 3-inch teenager, was spending a week at camp in the Georgia mountains. Because we had to pick our son up after camp, I had the bright idea of booking a honeymoon cabin in the same area to celebrate Hubby's birthday.

"Take a look at their website," I said to Hubby before reserving a cabin. "It looks nice. And it's not too far from the camp. We can go a few days beforehand."

"We will have two *entire* days. A-l-o-n-e," Hubby purred, rubbing his hands hungrily as if he were about to devour a side of beef. "I hope that bed is king size. Wait! Check out that 10-person Jacuzzi!" he exclaimed, his wheels already turning. Naturally, I imagined myself in traction following the christening of that fiberglass "den of iniquity."

On travel day, we headed north from our home in Southern Florida.

"Finally," sighed my depraved husband, as if I'd purposely deprived him of food or air for a month as we drove on the Florida Turnpike.

Hours later, we stopped for lunch. "Guess what? It's my birthday," he announced to our elderly waitress, adding a sly wink like some sex-starved teenager.

"Try to contain yourself," I whispered to him. I became more embarrassed as he rambled on to everyone within ear-shot about the "*horny*-moon" cabin that awaited us only 13 hours away.

It was when we passed an adult superstore and the "Ex-otic" Truck-Wash Cafe near the Georgia border that I real-ized things were a bit out of hand. Predictably, I was shocked when Hubby actually pulled into the parking lot.

"Oh, my God! What are we doing here?" I shrieked. We had zoomed past the sleazy establishment for more than 20 years but never had the pleasure of stopping—until then.

"You'll see," Hubby said, dashing inside while I sat hor-rified, slumping down in the car seat as hordes of truckers traipsed into this pole-dancing, biscuit-and-gravy serving, prophylactic emporium. Hubby emerged minutes later grin-ning like a Cheshire cat with an arsenal of X-rated God-knows-what.

"I bought you a surprise," he gushed, handing me an or-ange hooker nightie, complete with feathers and bells. Yes—tiny bells like the ones I used to string through my baby's shoe laces.

"Oh, my, flame resistant, too!" I sarcastically added.

"It'll come in handy while we're burning up the sheets," Hubby said, laughing. I pictured my tinkling bells announc-ing the impending boudoir three-alarm fire.

Unfortunately, between the snarling Atlanta traffic, spotty GPS service and the windy mountain roads, it was after midnight when we arrived at the secluded cabin for our first night of "amore." Ha! Some first night. The romance of the anticipated horny-moon cabin—with its bearskin rug, canopied bed, fireplace and oversized Jacuzzi—was totally lost on us as we collapsed, snoring and drooling, until noon.

"What would you like to do for your birthday—besides the obvious?" I teased my husband that morning, coffee in hand. "We don't get my baby until tomorrow and I'd like to see something while we're here, something besides the inside of this cabin."

Agreeing to the sightseeing adventure, Hubby was a man on a mission, zooming through our tourist activities in three hours flat.

"It might be nice to have our picnic *outside* the car," I said. Hubby zipped along the back roads while I balanced the cheeseboard on my lap and pulled the cork from the wine bottle with my teeth.

By three that afternoon, Hubby was ready to start some serious birthday celebrating. Poor Hubby. Whoever said good things come to those who wait has obviously never been on an 800-mile pilgrimage for birthday sex. Like a last-minute clemency call from the governor, Hubby's cellphone rang. He answered it while driving.

"So, if it's dislocated, they can just pop it back in, right? I think it would be best if he returns to camp to show the other boys he's fine."

*Uh oh. That doesn't sound good*, I said to myself.

"What's happened?" I asked Hubby, in a panic. My Mama Bear intuition kicked in as Hubby continued speaking with the scoutmaster. "Call us when you know something," he said, hanging up.

"He may have dislocated his shoulder. They're taking him to the hospital as a precaution. It's no big deal. Saw this all the time when I played football. He'll be fine," he shared, as if my baby had stubbed his toe on a daisy. "Hey, why don't we stop and get some Champagne for tonight?"

"What's wrong with you? My baby is in the ER! You get me to the hospital this instant!" I ordered.

"But, it's my birthday," he mumbled under his breath.

"Don't even go there!" I screamed.

We arrived at the hospital, and I did my best to keep a stiff upper lip while the doctor popped my baby's shoulder into place. Moments later, things were just short of lunacy—thanks to my two boys.

"This is the best shot e-v-e-r!" my baby yelled exuberantly, hopped up on pain meds.

Hubby repeated his cliché to anyone—conscious or not—in the ER. "You know, tomorrow is my birthday."

I resembled a dog chasing a boomerang, running back and forth, trying to shut them both up. Note to future self—next time we visit the ER, don't forget the insurance card, medical records and a big roll of duct tape.

I don't have to tell you that the news hit my husband like a brick when the doctor announced that not only could my baby not return to camp as Hubby had planned, but he couldn't be moved for the next 36 hours.

"No problem, we have a sofa bed in our cabin that's very comfortable," I responded. Hubby looked at me as if I were the devil.

"Are you sure?" Hubby questioned the doctor.

The doctor, scoutmaster and I stared at him, completely stunned.

"I'm sure the cot is quite comfortable in his tent at camp and that sling he's got on looks pretty sturdy. This storm will pass soon, too. You know tomorrow is my birthday and . . ."

I was appalled, as were the doctor, the nurses and the scoutmaster. They obviously didn't grasp the enormity of Hubby's plight. After all, he was the true victim in this tragedy—my long- suffering husband.

"Why don't you just lock him in a hot car," I said sarcastically.

Back at the cozy cabin for three, my precious baby snored comfortably on his sofa bed next to Hubby's bubbling hot tub and romantic roaring fire.

I almost felt sorry for Hubby. He did deserve an "A" for perseverance during his pitiful last-ditch effort to save his beloved X-rated birthday while we were in the ER. That was, until he said to me back at the cabin, "Perhaps tomorrow he could go to camp just for a few hours and complete some of his scout badges."

"Are you kidding me? He's not going anywhere!"

"But, it's . . ."

"Don't start," I snapped. "I know it's your birthday, and it's not what you planned, but you're going to have to move past this! I suggest you head down to the gas station and get yourself a six-pack and a beef jerky! You'll feel better. God knows I'll feel better. When you return, you can hop in the Jacuzzi with me. I'll even light these candles."

For a brief moment, I saw a glint of hope in his eyes until I killed it dead in an instant, donning my swimsuit and oversized T-shirt before sliding down into the gurgling water. "Hey, have you seen my razor?" I asked him.

With a look of total defeat, Hubby silently held up the atrocious nightie, the tag still attached, and dropped it back into the bag. He silently headed toward the front door.

"Honey, don't feel bad. There's always next year," I shouted over the whir of the jets as the door slammed behind him.

# A Couple of Drinks

by
Pat Nelson

All it takes is a few drinks to loosen me up and make me frisky. I guess that makes me either a cheap drunk or a loose woman. And I'm far too influenced by those playful love scenes on TV. My reenactments, especially after a couple of drinks, always lead to disaster.

One bitterly cold and snowy night, my husband, Bob, and I returned home from a Christmas party. Bob doesn't drink, so I'd had one for each of us. I must have stood under the party's mistletoe too long that evening, because by the time we arrived home, I was ready for some action, in spite of the late hour.

As soon as we walked into the house, I stripped off my clothes and left them in a heap under the Christmas tree. With twinkling eyes and a flirtatious smile, I said to Bob, "If you want your Christmas present early, meet me in the hot tub."

I took the plunge, and Bob joined me. Snow glistened around us. The night was still. Steam rose from the hot tub. Stars twinkled in a clear sky. Scooting over closer to me, expecting something special to happen, Bob didn't know I hadn't yet worked out the details of the gift I was about to present.

Suddenly, inspiration struck. I recalled something I had seen in a movie. "Come on," I said, "let's make love in the snow!"

Before either of us could reconsider, we plunged naked off the side of the hot tub into the snow, where we both began to moan. Fact: This wasn't fresh snow. It was topped with an icy crust that cut into us like knives. These were not moans of lust, but moans of pain.

Moments later, standing under a hot shower together, I asked Bob, "No hard feelings?"

"None," he assured me. I should have learned my lesson that night. There's a reason that, on TV, they say, "Don't try this at home."

But I had not learned a thing.

On a trip to Belize, after enjoying dinner and drinks with family, I felt giddy being with my loved one in paradise. My inebriated and now romantic state had set my imagination in motion. A sexy scene in my mind begged me to play the starring role.

Pheromones oozed from my smooth, tanned and oiled skin as Bob and I walked hand in hand toward the restaurant's exit. Looking out into the moonlit sky, Bob stepped down to the sand and offered his hand to help me down. I suddenly (meaning it was a surprise to me, too!) leaped into his arms and threw my legs around his waist. My 200-pound hunka-hunka burning love nearly brought him to his knees, right there at the restaurant door . . . because I had thrown out his back. The scene had worked better on TV.

Again that night, forgiving my foolish theatrics, Bob had no hard feelings.

And he no longer lets me watch R-rated movies or TV shows to get any new romantic ideas.

# The After-Sex Afghan

by
Sue Carloni

As newlyweds, we quickly settled into a weeknight routine. We would rush home from work, prepare dinner, do dishes, have sex in the bedroom, and then close the living room drapes and watch TV until bedtime. What made the TV cuddling extra special was that we would sit naked on the couch together, covered with the comfy, forest-green afghan my husband Kurt's grandmother had crocheted for our wedding gift.

Our weekend routine was much different from our weeknight norm. We dressed after our Saturday and Sunday sex, ready to take on whatever was on the agenda during our two days off. The afghan remained neatly folded on the couch.

One weeknight, after finishing our lovemaking, we snuggled under the afghan and watched one of our favorite TV programs. The doorbell rang. We looked at one another, wondering who would be coming over on a weeknight. We visited with friends and relatives only on the weekends.

If our car had been parked in the garage—and not the driveway, as it had been that night—we would have ignored the doorbell. Realizing our plight, we scrambled to the bedroom and threw on some clothes. By then, there was loud, relentless pounding on the front door. Kurt ran to open it while I checked the mirror to make sure my hair wasn't too messy.

Opening the door, there stood Kurt's parents, shivering in the cold Wisconsin winter. "What took you so long to answer the door?!" my mother-in-law demanded.

*How do you answer that question? How naïve is she?* I thought, now standing next to Kurt. We were both trying to catch our breath from the unexpected dressing and running around.

"Well, you see, we had great sex and were snuggling naked under Grandma's afghan and needed to quickly get dressed."

No! That wasn't the answer at all. Kurt made the excuse that he had just gotten out of the shower, and I was using the bathroom. Well, I guess my in-law's envisioning me taking a crap was better than their envisioning us naked on the couch after having sex.

His parents proceeded to sit on the couch, the very couch where our naked bodies had been lounging mere minutes before.

"Oh, I see you've been using Grandma's afghan," Kurt's mom commented, feeling the blanket's softness. "She'll be so pleased. I'll tell her how much you like it."

*Would Grandma like that?* I wondered. I imagined the horror on Grandma's face if she learned we referred to her gift as the "after-sex afghan."

We couldn't wait for Kurt's parents' surprise visit to end. Finally, they stood. As Kurt's mom reached for the doorknob, she suddenly turned and blurted, "Did we interrupt you two from sex?!"

Kurt's dad's face paled. My face turned red, while Kurt stared down at the floor, saying nothing.

"N-no," I stammered. The truth was, they had not interrupted sex. They had interrupted our intimate, relaxing-after-sex time under the after-sex afghan.

"We should have called ahead," his mom said.

"No, you don't need to do that," I said, even though I didn't mean it.

After they had driven away, we tore off our clothes and resumed our snuggling on the couch under the afghan—snuggling naked after having sex seemed to be a part of our lovemaking. And we didn't realize how important that was until it was disrupted.

Thanks, Mom and Dad.

# My Money's Worth

by
Ken McKowen

I stumbled out of the tiny house, through its unpainted and well-weathered wooden door, into a small dirt yard. Standing near a picket fence, I looked around. My groggy mind replayed fuzzy visions of a panting, moaning woman.

The Vietnam War was raging at the time, and I was in the Army, but stationed at a military base called "Hakata," located on the northwest coast of Kyushu, Japan. Walking back to the main street, which ran through the small Japanese village of Saitozaki, my memory was slowly becoming less fuzzy.

Our nights off-duty often resulted in an over consumption of Sapporo and Asahi beer and, even more dangerous, Nikka whiskey. Being only 19 years old and in a foreign land where a 50-yen taxi ride would deliver me to the small village where bars, alcohol and very friendly bar girls were plentiful, I was in heaven.

On one of our free nights, several of us headed into the local "ville" for a liquid dinner and perhaps a trip home with a bar girl. After all, we'd been paid and for a few thousand yen (about $6), you could drink yourself into a coma. And for 3,600 yen ($10), you could head home with one of the bar girls who offered after-hours entertainment. Like I said, it was heaven for a 19-year-old. And it was certainly a lot cheaper and more of a sure thing than a traditional date back in the States.

I'm certain the village's cute, young bar girls made more money than we did as they separated us from our pay by plying us with cheap booze and parading around in short skirts and tight-fitting, low-cut blouses. Since silicone implants weren't around yet, most of the girls had to work hard at creating any perception of actual cleavage. Still, our youth and horniness easily overshadowed any need for big boobs.

In one bar we frequented, there was a single exception to the cute and young ladies—an older woman. Our matronly barmaid was somewhere upward of age 40, which was ancient by our standards. She may have been the bar owner, or perhaps a holdover from the Korean War's G.I.s, but she was funny and friendly, and everyone loved talking and joking with her.

From here, the story becomes fuzzy, and it's not because I've tried to erase details of my first all-night encounter with one of those mysterious young Asian women of desirable repute, but rather because of the mind-numbing effects of the Nikka whiskey. To the contrary, I really wish I could remember more of the details because it was likely a fun and educational night. I do remember that the bar girls continued bringing us drinks, sitting on our laps and gathering tips. And I remember two in our party challenging each other to see who could chug the most from a bottle of tequila. The winner downed about three-fourths of the bottle and was still unconscious 24 hours later, but survived.

Those who were still standing when the bar closed headed back to base. But I, with my alcohol-encased brain, was led astray by one of the best-looking bar girls. As she and I left together, I heard jealous hoots and taunts from my friends, who were heading to the taxi stand by themselves, with only their hands for entertainment.

Her house was small—essentially a tiny living room with a tiny television and a tiny couch big enough for two. It was attached to a bedroom with no room for anything more than a bed. There was a "benjo"—a squat toilet—with no flushing capability, a U.S. luxury not yet common in Japan.

As far as the night of comely entertainment went, I still remember her asking for, and me paying, the 3,600 yen. I remember the soft bed and the real sheets, both much better than my Army bunk back on base. I do remember, or maybe I'm still fantasizing that after waking her up several times during the night to be sure I got my money's worth, she accused me of being an overly horny G.I. And I do remember she had cleavage, created by boobs bigger than any of the other bar girls' boobs in town . . . and bigger than any I had ever before personally befriended.

The one thing that still stands out in my mind over everything else is waking up in a daze the next morning. I rolled over and saw my hostess lying on her back, and those naked boobs—big naked boobs—that, rather than being firm and pointing straight up, hung over her sides. They partially covered a plump, semi-wrinkled body that belonged to the friendly and funny 40-something-year-old barmaid. To make matters worse, she had a smile on her face as she snored.

I quickly and quietly got out of bed, found my clothes and dressed, and then stumbled out of that weathered wood door. From that day on, I never again touched Nikka whiskey, and I made sure if I left with a bar girl, she was at least younger than my mother!

# A Very Long Week

by
Angela Miranda

My therapist gave me a challenge: try being single for a while.

I tried being truly single for the first time when I was 26. I'm 32 now. At that time, "single" meant I was not 100-percent, ready-to-get-married, permanently devoted to someone who would walk into traffic for me. It meant wearing my miniskirt and serving cocktails at a college bar, going on three dates a week, taking home easy targets and sometimes dating one for approximately 24 days.

But once the challenge was made, I committed to being done with men. No dates, no eHarmony, no more on-again, off-again drama with my Mexican lover or my Southern soldier. That meant no romance. I intended to keep this up for at least two weeks. Now, I didn't say "no sex." I couldn't bear to think about how that part of the equation would probably also be removed, unless I could figure out how to have sex after ending contact with all the people I liked to have sex with. Given that I was no longer into bar pickups or fumbling back to the hotel or the backseat, I convinced myself that the "still having sex" part would work itself out. This time, it would be the real thing—avoiding men by choice, sleeping alone and enjoying my own company.

After thinking it over, I thought better of the two-week thing. I committed to one week. My own company could prove to be intolerable.

Just as I embarked on this new adventure, my friend Brooke came to town for a visit and brought along her female cousin, who was married and had a two-year-old. This woman referred to herself as "more of a guy than her husband." She said this as if being a guy made her a better person, somehow more cool. I admired her self-esteem, but I didn't see the reasoning. I've had men tell me that I'm like a guy, too. But to me, it was as if they were saying, "You have very broad shoulders."

Shortly into our leisurely picnic, "Married Cousin" took a sip of her beer and began citing a study on the hormone oxytocin. She said that oxytocin is released into a woman's body when said woman has an orgasm.

I know this to be true, but I had to pause when I processed her exact words: "Since women release oxytocin after sex, it makes them more monogamous than men." I took her wild extrapolation to mean that she hadn't read any of Chelsea Handler's books. And I found myself thinking, "What the hell?"

Now I'm not trying to sound like a jerk, but I was a biology major in college. I also have a medical degree, so I know a bit about reproduction. Her statement was the most ass-contrived theory I had ever heard. Seriously. Look up "oxytocin" online or even in a medical database like PubMed. If you do, you will find all kinds of great information, such as how oxytocin is related to childbirth, breast-feeding and sexual arousal, and how, like lots of hormones, it affects brain function. It can increase trust between two members of a species and is part of "pair-bonding." Scientifically speaking, in the animal kingdom, "pair-bonding" means anything from "let's get married and raise babies together" to "let's drink wine and go down on each other." The reader should also note pair-bonding would never happen with only one orgasm.

I know there are way smarter people than I who study these things in earnest, but I caution: Before we go making predictions about how women will behave sexually, consider the big picture. Married Cousin is a case in point. Stunned to hear that others didn't think human sexuality was more complicated than her statement, I went dumb with silence and started piling tortilla chips into my mouth. That's what I do when I'm confused or ready to spout off.

As my companions continued to spout their pseudoscience, my mind wandered. Soon, I was engaged in my favorite mental challenge—dreaming up new *Saturday Night Live* characters. Per the theme of the day, my fantasy character was "Captain Oversimplify." In my imagination, he appeared magically atop our picnic table, in a puff of smoke, wearing his too-long red cape and bulging slightly out of his too-tight blue outfit. He proceeded to flit around, from me to Brooke and to Brooke's amateur-neurophysicist cousin, grasping our shoulders firmly one at a time, eyes wide with the anticipation of bestowing his brand of wisdom.

He said to me: "We can solve the energy crisis with light bulbs alone!"

To Brooke: "The only cause of cancer is too much stress!"

Finally, to Married Cousin: "Killer whales are actually very docile."

Obviously, Captain Oversimplify never wasted an opportunity to affirm your foregone conclusions.

Every time Captain Oversimplify made a profound statement, an imaginary room full of morons in my head gave him a standing ovation. I also pictured that room full of morons 30 years later, choking on carbon emissions in the scorching greenhouse heat and dying of lung cancer, which they obtained, of course, after breathing stress-free aromatherapy candles for three decades. At that point, the only thing that would save the world was the fact that none of these morons had any children left, because all of their pet killer whales had eaten their babies.

"I'm SERIOUS!" exclaimed Married Cousin. Startled, I choked on a tortilla chip, thus snapping me back to reality.

"What? Oh, right, I guess," I said, not sure what I had agreed to.

Later that evening, I called a friend for verification that I was not the only one who saw the subtle sexist bent in this earlier discussion. She was a librarian and, hence, very well read.

"Can you believe this cracked-out theory on monogamy?"

I asked her.

"Yeah, I mean, it makes evolutionary sense," she responded. "Men like to spread their seed and women like to mate with the most protective member of the species." I was baffled by her post-feminist summary of mating rituals, even though her tone was very matter-of-fact.

Double "What the hell?" Sure, females want to feel protected by those stronger than they are. Who doesn't? But would they perhaps want to mate—or just touch—for any number of reasons? Maybe they want to mate because they're ovulating. Maybe they want to spread certain genes they find attractive. Maybe they want to increase their odds of pregnancy by mating with whoever has a penis. Maybe they're seeking pleasure or closeness or just another orgasm. And maybe the thought ends there. We just don't know.

But as long as everyone around me wants to be a neuroscientist and reach back to our evolutionary roots for explanation, maybe we should think about our animal cousins. Some gorilla females prefer to live with other females and mate with just one male, only occasionally, when they feel like it. The bonobo chimpanzees, who share 98.7 percent of their DNA with humans, like to have sex with any other bonobo, anywhere, all the time. Their more immediate relatives—we human beings—can just as easily be bisexual polygamists as join in on a threesome or orgy. I take it these people don't have oxytocin?

Now consider me. Depending on the phase, I have found myself either wanting to sleep with a different man every day or with no one ever again. Compared to the average woman my age, I don't think I'm much of a player. I can still name them all, and even count them. At the same time, I'm no stranger to the occasional threesome or orgy fantasy.

All I'm saying is that if we want to believe one single hormone can predict the stereotyped behavior of all 3.5 billion human females, I won't buy it. I won't buy it because if I sit alone at home at night, with nothing but these thoughts to keep me company, it's gonna be a very long week.

CHAPTER THREE

# Oooopppssss!

Oh, no—you didn't!

# The Special Blue Pill

by
Christine Cacciatore

As I stood in the bathroom putting in my contact lenses, I suddenly heard my husband running down the hall toward me.

"What is this?!" he asked, holding out his open hand. Thinking it was a receipt or a bill, I quickly thought of a good excuse for whatever it was I had spent money on.

I was wrong. In his hand was the usual collection of vitamins, supplements and prescriptions people of our age take every morning—after the final cup of coffee, but before the inevitable morning-paper reading in the "office."

"What is what?" I asked after looking closer at the array of pills in his hand.

"This! Is this one of my . . . *special pills*?" he asked, eyebrows raised.

Our normal multivitamins were red. However, we had

run out of them a week ago. While shopping, I had grabbed the first replacements I saw—"One Daily, Men's 50+." As a nod to our age, the pharmaceutical company had colored them a pretty dove gray, a thoughtful match to the color of our hair.

The one my husband was concerned about, however, seemed to have received an extra shot of FD&C Blue No. 2, thus the reason he was so alarmed. It resembled *the other* type of blue pill, the kind one would take if he were going to . . .

Have you ever seen a Viagra commercial? The guy takes one of those blue happy pills then you see the couple flirting and kissing while playing the best damn Scrabble game of their entire freakin' lives. Or they're washing the car together, soaping seductively while shooting each other looks that say, "we're-so-gonna-get-it-on" as a Barry White song plays in the background.

If your hubby has ever used one of those pills, you know that the . . . um . . . *result* is a real eye-opener, a "Stand back, woman! This thing could be dangerous" kind of an eye-opener. I mean, you pretty much have to beat that thing into submission once it's had a taste of sapphire magic. Believe me, I know whereof I speak, and people, we do not waste the enchanted pills, am I right?

I finished putting my other contact in, which was hard (pun intended) while my whole body shook with laughter.

"Are you serious?" I giggled. "Do you really think I'm going to put one of those in your morning pill box as a joke? Pretty expensive joke, considering I could swap one on the black market in exchange for our mortgage payment. Besides, the Packers are playing the Bears this afternoon, and you're not even going to be here—you'll be at the bar with the boys."

Suddenly, the thought of him being stuck at the bar under the influence of one of those pills was hilarious to me. "How would you even get out of the bar without someone seeing your condition?" I asked him. "Seriously, you could hurt someone. On the upside, that thing would hold the door open for you."

He followed my lady-logic. "If it *were* one of those pills, I'd have to come home," he countered, "during *halftime*." He wiggled his eyebrows at me.

I was unmoved. "Pah! You'd come home to a note and an empty house, Romeo, because I'm going shopping this afternoon. That would put you in a pretty awkward position, wouldn't it? A party in your pants but no one 'comes,'" I said, making air quotes with my fingers.

"Real funny," he said. "Although I wouldn't see the note first." He leaned against the doorframe and smiled.

"Oh? And why not?"

"Because if you *had* slipped me one of those wonder pills," he said, pointing downward, "this thing would beat me home by at least 10 minutes."

# Whipped Cream Dreams

by
Julie Hatcher

On my wedding day, the snow-white magnolia trees were in full bloom, as well as my love for my Prince Charming. However, our ride into the sunset immediately after the reception shook our senses and compromised our claim of a picture-perfect wedding.

We waved goodbye to family and friends, and my new husband started the car. Pulling away, he flipped on the A/C. Suddenly, flour flew out of the air vents, followed by a stench that reeked to high heaven . . . fish!

Rounding a corner, my husband slammed on the brakes, got out of the vehicle, opened the hood and with his bare hands, catapulted the cooked sardines he'd found onto the street. My hero had rescued us from the pranks of naughty relatives. Gathering his composure, he got back into the driver's seat. We continued on our "Happily-Ever-After" journey, smelling like sardines.

We arrived at our honeymoon suite a few hours later. With its oversized whirlpool tub in the center of the room, it was the perfect place for my fantasy to become a reality.

Just like the cute little old lady in the movie *Patch Adams*, the one who dreamed of swimming in a pool full of spaghetti, I dreamed of swimming in a whirlpool tub full of whipped cream!

My husband, a willing accomplice, and I drove to the grocery store, grabbed a cart and rolled to the dairy aisle. I wiped the shelf clean of all brands of the delicious whipped topping. Counting 13 cans at the checkout counter, I wondered if it would be enough. I'd never made such a hefty purchase of the stuff and felt guilty, like a cat that'd just swallowed 13 baby birds. I reasoned that if other customers wanted dessert topping, tubs of whipped topping were available in the freezer section. We exited the store with only a minor smirk from the cashier.

When we returned to our room, the gigantic tub stared me in the face like a blank canvas waiting to be transformed into a work of art. I envisioned a fluffy cumulus-cloudlike mass filling the tub and folding over the top rim. My husband and I would be the subjects in what I coined, "The Garden of Whipped Cream Delights!"

Gauging the cleanliness of the tub's bowl, I purified the space with warm running water in preparation for the baptismal. My husband, an eager-to-get-the-job-finished guy, began spraying a can of whipped topping, unleashing the precious sacrament before I could say, "Wait!" His spew amounted to no more than a softball-sized mound, followed by sprays of air that splattered the sphere into an ellipse then scattered into cirrus-cloud wisps.

"No! You released it too fast!" I scolded.

I attempted to expertly point the nozzle in proximity to the surface and carefully coaxed the foam out of its package. Within seconds, air shot out, so I shook it and jiggled it . . . upside down, right side up then sprayed some more to ensure I pulled out the last drop! My husband joined in, but the 13 cans of wonderfulness only covered the bottom of the tub, much to my chagrin. Resolutely, I settled for whatever this batch could give me.

As I stood there staring at our fluffy, sugary mounds in the bottom of the tub, I sighed. Then we laughed. I concluded that our demise would make for good conversation, even though my bucket-list item remained unchecked. Next time, my plans would be tighter and my pockets deeper. We bared all and sank into our mini-masterpiece.

We had our kicks, spinning, sliding and not getting any traction and too little friction. As the creaminess dissipated, the stickiness made its premiere, and my desire for clean skin again sharpened. Retiring to a tiled shower stall large enough to accommodate five people made me question the history of previous exploits in that room.

With our event complete and our aspirations somehow appeased, we returned to look at our now-milky island of paradise. I'd not considered how to clean up the mess after the mayhem. Filling the tub with water, clumps of fat stood on end, not budging and refusing to go down the drain. I couldn't imagine what would have happened if we'd reached the level of enjoyment and mass that I dreamed of. That's when I truly appreciated that we had only 13 cans of goo to clean up.

Mopping up the stubborn little devils of cream, we employed every towel and washcloth in the room. Paper towels would've been the amicable choice, avoiding any possibility of a housekeeper holding her nose and saying, "What in God's name did these cows do to these towels?" I'm sure the generous number of cans found in the trash could at least account for the odor, while the number of cows who actually occupied the room could only be left to her own embellished fantasy.

The next morning, we boarded a plane to the Grand Cayman. As I settled into my seat, the odor of soured milk poured over me like a ton of bricks. I sniffed my husband's hair and clothes. He sniffed mine. Our whipped cream extravaganza still lingered, soured on the surface, but all sweet in-between. As co-conspirators in the great whipped-topping experiment, we smiled and laughed. For better or for worse, we harbored a secret and the scent of sweetly soured dreams.

# The Neighbors

by
Carol Commons-Brosowske

Have you ever wanted to unmeet someone?

Davis and Sue lived behind us for more than 20 years. We were never what I'd call best friends although we enjoyed chatting and being with them at neighborhood gatherings. They were a nice, friendly couple. Since we saw them frequently—either working in the yard or driving past—we would swap stories on occasion about our families and juicy neighborhood gossip. And we were always there for one another if we needed to borrow a cup of sugar or milk. It was a good relationship all the way around.

I recall the day I told Sue we were expecting our first grandchild. While I was unloading groceries from my car, Sue pulled into her driveway. We waved and began exchanging a few words. She seemed genuinely excited about me being a first-time grandmother. "I was just going to take our port-a-crib to the resale shop. Would you like it instead?"

I jumped at the chance of getting a crib for free and walked to her car. A self-admitted cheapskate, I was always on the hunt for bargains. I'm especially happy to accept free items any day of the week!

Sue gathered up her purse then said, "Go on into my house and take a look. It's right beside the kitchen counter." I opened up the door and walked in, with Sue right behind me. Their house was an open-concept style, so the minute you walked into the back door, you were in the kitchen facing the family room.

As I took a few steps inside the house, I saw Davis in his recliner in the family room. The chair sat at an angle in the corner. Just as I was about to call out a friendly greeting, I noticed he was, shall I say, "preoccupied."

There he sat, naked as a jaybird! He was wearing headphones and was having the time of his life. His chair rocked back and forth and wiggled from side to side all at the same time. His arm was flailing up and down faster than a speeding bullet. It didn't take a genius to figure out he was masturbating. Because of the headphones, Davis hadn't a clue that his wife and neighbor were watching.

With his eyes rolled back into his head as his pleasure spewed out right in front of us, he didn't hear Sue screaming, "Davis, what in the hell are you doing?!"

All I could think of was to get the hell out of a most precarious sticky situation. I simply said, "I'll get the crib another time. I really need to finish unloading my car." Head down, I whirled around and after several attempts at trying to get the doorknob to turn, I made my escape, running as fast as my 61-year-old legs could go. The last thing I saw was Sue standing there wide-eyed and thunderstruck. I'd never known that a person could turn white as a sheet and red as a beet all at the same time, but that's exactly what she did.

Back on my own turf, I bolted into the house screeching for my husband. "Oh! My! Gosh! You're never going to believe what just happened!" I explained what I'd witnessed, and he laughed so hard I thought he might fall on his face. I must admit that I've giggled more than once thinking about that spectacle.

As humiliated as I'm sure they both were, I did feel much empathy for poor Sue. Mercy, how embarrassed she must have been. I can only imagine what took place between them after I abruptly left. I'd have given a million bucks to have been a fly on the wall for that conversation.

Since that day, things have never been quite the same between us. Simple nods and waves are all that remain. I ended up buying my own crib, and I will now go to the store looking like death warmed over for any emergency items rather than borrowing anything from them. I fear I could end up seeing something much worse should I dare to darken their door again.

Will I ever be able to get that vision out of my head? I seriously doubt it. I often wonder what I'd have done if the roles had been reversed. My answer is always the same. I would have moved clear across town, hoping never to run into either of them again. If, for some reason, I ever do encounter Davis up close, I'll be polite. But if he expects a handshake, it just ain't gonna happen, come hell or high water.

# It's Just a Penis

by
Bobby Barbara Smith

"Well, happy birthday to me!" I muttered as I drove to work. No days off for this single mom. I had three kids to feed, a house payment to make and all that goes with those scenarios. But I didn't linger long in my pity party. I felt blessed to have a job, and while it was hard work and long hours, it paid the bills.

"Good morning," I said to my co-workers as I arrived at the high-end dry cleaners where I worked. I noticed some nudging and smiles floating among them, but my sense of duty called and I didn't have time to think much about it.

It was a busy morning, and I focused on customers, forgetting about the whispers and giggles until one of the girls called me to the back. "Bobby, can you come here for a minute?" Katie asked, flashing an evil smile as I walked past her. In back, my co-workers gathered around a white box and grinned like hyenas.

"We wanted to get you something for your birthday, so we pooled our money for a gift. We know you don't have anyone special in your life, so we thought this would add a little spice to your day," another co-worker said, motioning to the box.

My co-workers were an eclectic, street-smart, fun-loving group of people. So no telling what they had bought me. As I approached the box, the guys hung back while the gals practically foamed at the mouth, demanding I open my gift NOW! I looked at their impish faces and knew something foul was inside it. But there was no way to escape.

I flipped open the lid and found myself staring at a huge penis cake, complete with an erection and hairy balls! I could feel red creeping up my neck and flooding my face while my devilish friends doubled over with laughter. Even though I was a divorced mom in my late 30s, I had led an extremely sheltered life. I obviously knew what a penis was—I had three children. But a cake? Who would make such a thing? And who would eat it?

"We don't have a knife. You'll just have to grab a chunk and eat it," a male voice said. I recognized it as belonging to one of the pressers who had hit on me more than once.

"Creep!" I responded. I refused to look up at his smirking face, but staring at the thing in front of me wasn't helping matters, either.

"It's just a penis, Bobby," Katie said, stopping her laughing long enough to interject. "Surely you remember."

"Vaguely!" I threw Katie a warped smile, determined she and the rest of the group weren't going to get the best of me.

I was relieved when the lobby bell signaled a customer entering, but the relief was short-lived. It was our boss, and he was walking toward us in the back of the shop.

"He can't see this!" I screamed. I slammed the lid shut and shoved the box under the worktable. My giggling co-workers scattered to their respective workstations.

"Hey, Bobby. What's up?" the boss asked me. Loud snorts came from across the room.

"We've been busy," I said, trying to act normal and hoping he wouldn't notice my red face and snickering co-workers.

"That's good. Oh, happy birthday. I chipped in on the gift. Hope they got you something nice." He paused at my worktable and smiled.

*Does he know?* I thought to myself. *No way! He would never do that!*

"A cake . . . they got me a cake," I stammered as I glanced at the box, praying he wouldn't want to see it.

"Cool! Wish I could stay and have a piece, but I'm late as it is." He was barely out the door when laughter burst out. I struggled to hide the smile creeping across my face, but it was futile. I gave up and joined in the laughter. The boss . . . the cake . . . his comments . . . it kept us all in stitches for the rest of the shift.

Since no one wanted any cake, I was stuck with it. *Guess I'll have to take that thing home. I can't leave it here.*

As I drove, I wondered how I would hide it from the kids. My daughter was going home with a friend after school, but the boys would hit the kitchen first thing, starving, as usual.

Once home, I shoved the box into the freezer, thinking it would be safe there. That's when I decided to take a shower. It had been quite the day.

Turning off the shower faucet, I heard my boys come home and then rustle around in the kitchen for food. I dried off, threw on some comfy clothes and headed in their direction.

"Is that what I think it is?" I heard my 12-year-old ask his older brother, followed by dual scoffing.

"Man, look at the size of it!" the 14-year-old exclaimed.

I rounded the corner to see the cake box on the counter and both boys staring into it, giggling like girls.

"Boys, I put that in the freezer for a reason. But now that you've seen it . . . it was a birthday joke my co-workers played on me," I explained as casually as possible.

"Is it edible? I'm hungry!" my oldest asked, well over the surprise.

But the younger one still stared at the cake. "I have a question, Mom. Is that normal size?" he said, pointing at it. He had a look of grave concern on his face.

"No, it's not normal size," I assured him. I giggled a bit then put on my serious mom face. "It's exaggerated, like most stories you'll hear on the subject. Just remember, size isn't important.

"Wait 'til I tell the guys! They won't believe it!" he then said, his eyes lighting up with excitement.

I shot him down fast. "Don't you dare breathe a word of this to anyone—do you hear me?" I shuddered at the thought of my cake story circulating around their school.

"What's the big deal, Mom?" asked big brother. Wise beyond his years, he always had a way of putting things into perspective. "It's just a penis."

# Twice in One Day

by
Renee Hughes

"How exciting!" I said when my husband announced we were both invited to the church's annual planning retreat. This trip would be a rare overnight stay without the children, and I was thrilled. My husband and I had traveled on business in the past, but one of us always stayed home with the kids.

Arrangements were quickly made for a relative to watch the children. Packing my overnight bag, I included skimpy lingerie and a fresh tube of K-Y Jelly, hoping for an evening to remember. The retreat was nestled in a serene, wooded area which would provide minimal outside interruptions and would be oh-so romantic.

After dinner and team-building exercises with the other church members, my husband and I returned to our room. My heart rate raced with anticipation. While my husband fluffed the pillows and lay down on the bed to read, my preparation activities went unnoticed. I hung a dress for the meeting the next day to let the wrinkles fall out and finished unpacking my suitcase. Then I sneaked the lingerie into the bathroom under the guise of setting up my toiletries and makeup bags for the following day.

After donning my nightie, I touched up my lipstick, sprayed on his favorite perfume and tidied my hair. I turned the knob and barely opened the door when gentle snoring floated through the crack. With his devoted effort to prepare for the meeting, on top of a difficult Friday at work and the drive to the retreat, my husband had exhausted himself. Tiredness canceled my planned evening of bliss.

I slept in the next morning and arose with barely enough time to shower, wash my hair, grab a piece of fruit and arrive at the first session. When I got out of the shower, I searched my travel bag for hair gel, but there was none. I dumped its contents onto the counter, touching and pushing aside each item to make sure I hadn't overlooked it, but still nothing. Panic set in—without hair gel, my fine, naturally-curly shoulder-length hair rivaled that of the Greek goddess Medusa.

Since the nearest store was miles away, I couldn't run out and buy more hair gel. Now late for the first session, I scampered up and down the hall—wet head and all—to ask if anyone else from our group had brought hair product. As I made my inquiries, my hair began to dry and grew in voluminous and scary jagged corkscrews.

Not finding any hair gel, I returned to our room and contemplated hiding there until we left that evening. But that wouldn't work as we had to check out before lunch then return to the meeting. I was doomed.

I desperately searched my travel bag again, but no hair gel magically appeared. Frustrated, I turned and accidently knocked something from the bathroom counter onto the floor—the K-Y Jelly. Smiling, I dialed back my alarm and asked myself, *How different can jelly be from hair gel?*

I slathered a dollop of the jelly onto my now barely damp hair. Using the blow dryer on the lowest setting possible, I did my hair. It worked! With sex lubricant on my head, I sauntered into the church's group meeting. The rest of that day, I sported a mischievous grin *and* perky hair!

On our trip home, I admitted to my husband I had put K-Y Jelly on my hair. His eyes grew wide, and he asked, "What? Why didn't you tell me earlier?"

"I didn't want to distract you from your mission today," I answered. "Later after the children are turned in, I want to use the lubricant as intended per the directions on the tube."

Smiling to myself about my sexy invite, I thought, *Yes, she does use jelly—and twice in one day!*

# The Day
# I Had Balls

by
Amanda Mushro

When I was a freshman in college, I self-diagnosed some uncomfortable itching in my nether region as a yeast infection. Since I was an independent woman out on my own—just kidding, my parents were footing the bill for me to live it up in college—I marched myself to the nearest pharmacy to fix my ailing va-jay-jay.

When I looked at the over-the-counter yeast infection remedies, I found several brands claiming to cure that not-so-comfy-feeling "down there." But it was the number that caught my eye. One brand had a seven-day treatment, another a five-day treatment, and another, a one-day treatment. Clearly, the one-day treatment was the way to go. *Who would suffer from this crap for five days—or worse, seven?* I said to myself, answering, *Fools, that's who!*

After making my purchase of the one-day treatment, I headed back to the dorms to begin the healing process.

About an hour after the application of the medication, things started to happen—and not in a good way.

At first, I grew even more uncomfortable and felt as if someone had turned up the heat in my dorm room. Then I realized I was sweating because things were getting hot in the lady garden. Clearly, something wasn't right.

Needing to inspect this burning issue, I headed to the bathroom I shared with the other females on my dorm floor. Dropping my drawers, I checked out my girly bits, which led to the shock of my life. My who-ha had transformed into balls!

Yes, friends. Balls. The swelling was so bad that everything in my bikini area was barely recognizable. Horrified by my new appendages, I let out a scream that echoed the white walls of the communal bathroom.

My roommate rushed in. "What's wrong?!" she asked, pushing open the stall door.

"Something isn't right, but I don't want to show you," I answered, attempting to close my legs. *How do guys close their legs with these things?*

I was so humiliated, but I knew I had to show someone. Closing my eyes and taking a deep breath, I used the walls of the stall to push myself up. Then I braced myself for her reaction. *Maybe it's not as bad as I think . . .*

When my roommate saw my new accessories, she let out a yelp and cried, "What did you do to her?" That's when I knew it was as horrible as I had thought. Honestly, in times like this, it's bad enough when you, alone, are freaking out. But when you call in backup and they panic too, that means the shit is real.

I struggled to pull up my pants then wobbled back to my room. Clearly, I needed some medical attention. But because I was a freshman, I didn't have a car. *What am I going to do?* I could barely walk, so hiking it over to Student Health was not an option. *Seriously, how do guys walk with these things?*

My new appreciation for the male species being able to walk a straight line was cut short when I realized I had to resort to calling my only emergency contact with a car—my older brother, who was a senior at the same university.

Here's the gist of my phone call to him: "So, you know how you always wanted a brother, but you were stuck with me? Good news! I have balls now! I may be morphing into a dude. I need to go to the emergency room to make sure everything is cool down there. Can you come pick me up?"

After 15 minutes of my brother laughing his ass off at my aliment, he finally drove me to the ER so they could check out my balls. The humiliation was not to end there as my brother helped me to waddle into the ER only to be seen by the hottest intern I have ever laid eyes on. *Really? A hot doctor? You're just messing with me now, universe. Right?*

Dr. Mc Hotty: "Hi there, I'm Dr. Mc Hotty. What seems to be the problem?"

Me: "Well, Doc. Can I call you "Doc?" It would seem that I have balls."

Dr. Mc Hotty: "Balls?"

Me: "Yes. Balls. I grew them today and would like to get rid of them ASAP. Sort of like neutered."

Dr. Mc Hotty: "Well, let's check out your balls."

Me: "Only if you buy me dinner first." (Insert smile and a wink, trying to distract from the fact this gorgeous doctor was going to check out the horror movie that is my vagina.)

After further inspection, Dr. Mc Hotty prescribed lots of Benadryl to calm everything down, and he told me to not have sex for a few days. I think he added the no-sex part because I had attempted to flirt with him and tried to slip him my number multiple times. Yeah, not one of my finest moments, but the man was adorable, and he had already seen me partially naked. Why not?

The good doctor sent me home with Benadryl and a pat on the back. I'm sure my balls made for some awesome conversation at the nurse's station.

I'm happy to say that after this traumatic event and some Benadryl, my balls disappeared that very night and my lady bits returned to their normal size. I have sworn off self-diagnosing and yeast infection medicines since then. However, I am adamant on using this story as a cautionary tale to any of my friends that feel the need to clear up some itching on their own. I've become an urban legend in the yeast-infection world. Go for the seven-day treatment. Better yet, go to a doctor. And hope for a hot doctor. He'll take your mind off your balls.

# Masterstrokes

by
Stephen Hayes

In 1983, I had a stroke of genius. Or so I thought.

I was unhappy with my career in retail and ready for a change. One evening after a grueling day of peddling hardware, I picked up one of my wife's decorating magazines and noticed that a few of the rooms on display had reproductions of famous paintings—not prints, but high-caliber oil copies.

I had a degree in fine arts and decided to try to make a go of it as a painter. Creating copies for rich clients could be a lucrative way to start. If somebody wanted Thomas Gainsborough's *Blue Boy* hanging above their fireplace and couldn't convince the Huntington Library in Southern California to part with it, they could call me and I'd come up with the next best thing—a superbly painted copy. And if they wanted Thomas Lawrence's famous *Pinkie* hanging on the opposite wall, I could paint that, as well.

Before launching my business, I needed to come up with a snappy name. I chose "Masterstrokes," which, I believed, said it all. I checked the department of licenses, permits and registrations for my state to be certain nobody was already using the name. Learning it was available, I licensed it and had business cards printed up. I bought an ad in the *Yellow Pages*, mailed out flyers to local interior decorators and waited for the calls to pour in. I had a good feeling about this venture and couldn't help but wonder what I'd be asked to copy first, maybe a Canaletto or, perhaps, a Rembrandt.

But things didn't go as planned.

No art lovers or interior decorators called to offer me fat commissions to replicate old masters. The calls I received all came late at night. The first call went something like this:

*Ring. Ring. Ring.*

"Er . . . hello?" I asked, trying to shake the cobwebs from my brain.

"Hi. How you doing?"

"I'm doing all right. Who is this?"

"I'm someone calling to inquire about your services."

"My services?"

"Yes. This is Masterstrokes, isn't it?"

"Yes it is."

"Good, good. That's why I'm calling. What do you charge?"

"Well, it depends on how big a job it is."

"Believe me when I say I have a big job."

"That's wonderful. Some things are harder to do than others."

"You're absolutely right, and what I have in mind is really hard . . . exceptionally hard."

"Great. There's nothing I can't do. I went to college to learn my craft and I'm not embarrassed to admit I'm very good."

"I believe you."

"I also offer a money-back guarantee. If you aren't satisfied, you pay nothing."

"Really?"

"You can go anywhere and get the cheap stuff."

"That's been my experience."

"I deal in quality."

"Great! You know, my wife is interested in getting in on this, too. Would she be extra?"

"Extra?"

My wife was now awake and listening in. After a few minutes, she looked at me as if I had "moron" embossed on my forehead. She reached over to disconnect the call.

"Masterstrokes, my ass!" she mumbled as she struggled to get back to a night of fitful sleep.

Neither of us would sleep well until the new phone book arrived without an ad for Masterstrokes.

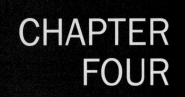
CHAPTER
FOUR

# What's the Speed Limit of Sex?

It's 68. At 69, you blow a rod.

# Coitus Calamitous

by
Juliette Lemieux

During weekend coffee klatches, my girlfriends share their sexual encounters, interludes, trysts and liaisons—all words laden with romance and sensuality. Whenever I share my stories, I tend to gravitate toward the words "incident" and "accident." To be honest, misfortune has plagued me since childhood, and why I thought trouble would stop short of the bedroom door, I do not know.

At 22, my boyfriend, Grant, bought a new Buick LeSabre, white and pristine.

"Hop in, Juliette," Grant said. "Let's take it for a spin."

And we did. Then he had a better idea. "Let's break it in." He tossed me a wicked smile.

As we raced down the highway, I unbuckled my seat belt, unzipped his shorts and lowered my head to his lap. His moans and groans were soon replaced with the ping of loose gravel, the screeching of metal on metal and the shattering of glass.

Once the car stopped flipping like a Nevada tumbleweed in September, I had not only landed in the back of the car, but I was also sitting on the roof, which now served as the floor of the vehicle. The doors had caved in from hitting both the guardrail and the ground so many times that they wouldn't open. Stunned, we sat in silence, listening to an ambulance approaching from a distance.

"Well," Grant said, "that was different."

I peered out to see a clan of people running down the embankment toward the car.

"Are your pants zipped?" I called from the back.

"What the hell kind of question is that?" he said, using his shirt sleeve to wipe a trickle of blood from his head.

I wasn't going out with a stained reputation. "Just checking." I pointed outside the car. "Look."

"Oh, shit." He quickly tucked and zipped before we crawled through a broken window to greet our rescuers.

"Wow," one of the men said. "The way your car left the roadway, my wife and I feared the worst. We saw the whole thing."

*Crap*, I thought.

"The whole thing?" I asked, embarrassed.

"Yeah." The man shielded his eyes from the sun then said, "But we thought there was only one person in the car."

Relief settled in. "Oh," I said, "I had the seat leaned back. You know . . . resting."

"Yeah," Grant added. "And stupid me, I had to go and

fall asleep, too."

*Good thinking, Grant.*

My head hurt, and I started to sway.

The helpful man grabbed my arm. "You two should take a seat until the ambulance comes. By the looks of the car, you're lucky to be alive."

The car was totaled, along with our libido. After interrogation by the police officer, an ambulance transported us to the hospital for evaluation, but not before we received a standing ovation from a crowd that had assembled on the nearby overpass to gawk at the wreckage. I knew the applause was for our survival, not for my cosmic fellatio technique, but I couldn't help but wonder if any other woman had ever made the earth tremble in such a way.

For the next several years, bad luck continued to lurk about. Like the time my husband, Lucas, and I took a day off work. No kids. No plans. No worries. After lunch, Lucas tossed me the I-want-to-do-you look, and who was I to resist?

We headed to our favorite place—the shower—for a splash of foreplay in anticipation of an afternoon of pleasure.

Lucas stripped and began adjusting the water temperature while I shed my jeans and sweater, eager to join him. He had flirted with me all morning: a caress when he passed me in the hallway on his way to get coffee, a hungry glance overtop the newspaper across the breakfast table, a playful kiss while I washed the dishes at the sink, a compliment while I dressed for the day. He was a smart man, knowing that desire begets desire.

I spread two towels on the bathroom countertop, so we could quickly dry each other before slipping into the nearby bed to extend our lovemaking. He climbed inside the bathtub and stood underneath the showerhead. I watched as the water trickled down his chest, wet and glistening. The sight heightened my arousal.

He motioned for me. "Come on in. The water's fine," he teased.

Slipping behind him, I drew the curtain, sequestering us in our afternoon hideaway. I pressed against his backside, forming suction between us. Not that I minded being glued to him—his body folding neatly into mine. I could have stayed there all day. His hands reached behind me, grabbing my cheeks while I blindly groped for the bar of soap on the shelf above. I lathered my hands and slid them across his chest, slowly working my way around his body.

"Your turn," Lucas said, as he motioned for the soap, ready to caress me.

When I turned away from the water and toward the back of the shower, my ass hit Lucas in the thigh. His knees gave way and caught the lip of the bathtub, which sent him soaring out of the shower. Years as a college gymnast played to his advantage—a handspring, followed by a somersault, spared him from crashing into the bathroom cabinetry, which could have resulted in a head injury. Lord knows, I didn't need to explain another sex accident to the police.

Still soapy and shaken, Lucas climbed back in to rinse off. "Jesus," he said, slapping me on the ass. "You need to register that thing as a deadly weapon."

A few months later, Calamity checked in with us at a hotel in Toledo. After dinner and cocktails, Lucas and I went back to the hotel for a night of lovemaking. In the throes of passion, I turned and kneeled on all fours, and Lucas grabbed the faux headboard mounted to the wall to steady himself and provide leverage as we rocked back and forth, doggy style. The headboard soon gave way and crashed onto the bed.

"Mother f_ _ _ _ r," Lucas said, stopping short of climax.

Drywall and screws littered the sheets.

We heard someone yell, "What the hell was that?" from the adjoining room, and we began laughing.

"Well, alrighty, then," I said. I crawled out of the bed, dusting off my breasts and thighs.

"Talk about *headboardus interruptis*," Lucas said as we cleaned off the bed so we could sleep.

The next morning, I pointed to the wooden piece propped against the wall. "Do you think they'll charge us?"

Lucas shook his head and marched to the front desk. I followed, but let him do the talking.

"We'd like to request a room change," Lucas started. "The headboard that was mounted to the wall fell off and nearly killed my wife in her sleep last night."

I peered out from behind him and nodded my head.

"Oh, my gosh," the clerk said. "Let me get my manager."

After Lucas had convinced the manager that their faulty carpentry nearly ended in tragedy, we were provided not only a suite, but also complimentary meals for the rest of our stay.

These days, Lucas and I remain optimistic about our

sex life. But given my past debacles, we refrain from using ropes or pulleys and chains or whips. Adventurous orgasms are nice but, most importantly, we want to make it out alive.

# Spitfire

by
Cappy Hall Rearick

Being a young virgin in the 1970s was different. Girls in my generation used to brag they'd done it when they hadn't.

My girlfriends and I claimed to be virgins long after we should have just shut up about it. We never seemed to tire of proclaiming it, as though it were a badge of honor worn with a long face and a hopeful heart. Truth be told, none us liked the idea of containing our hormones any longer than necessary, but neither did we want to risk having the reputation of being easy.

The day I left for college, however, I told myself that life was about taking risks, embracing exceptions. If I intended to live a full life, I would need to take some chances.

I knew at an early age that I would be a writer. Ordinary housewives might dream about exciting escapades, but authors lived them. Dolly Domestic did not occupy a place in my future, but "Brenda Star—Ace Reporter," did. I planned to zip from one spine-tingling experience to the other, much like my heroine comic book star reporter.

The road to my first carnal adventure began soon after my freshman year in college. That was the night Beaumont Bellingham popped my proverbial cherry, and the earth moved inside his Triumph Spitfire sports car.

Beaumont drove down a deserted road on the edge of town, pulled the Spitfire over to the side of the road, turned the motor off and yanked up the emergency brake that separated the two seats. After giving some thought to the position of the brake and to what he had in mind, he jerked the brake handle back into the down position. In retrospect, it was a good move.

We sat in the dark for a while not saying a word, both of us burning up with hormonal anxiety. Before long, Beaumont put his hand on my left knee and began to make little circles on it with his thumb. Then he started talking.

Beaumont had an opinion on almost every subject, which is why people often said he was cerebral. That night, for some crazy reason, he babbled about his theory regarding the fallacy of socialism or capitalism. I can't remember which, but I do remember his thumb circling my inner thigh, moving higher and higher with each revolution.

That morning before our date, I determined not to put off my sexual initiation another day. It was to be the first and perhaps the biggest of what I thought of as my life experiences. I chose a flared skirt with a loose fitting sweater to wear that night since I didn't just fall off the back of a turnip truck. I had been reading romance magazines since I was

13 years old and I had learned a thing or two between the moanings and the mornings.

Back then, we sneak-smoked regular cigarettes because we didn't know about the funny kind. They were Pall Malls—or rather "Pell Mells," as my cerebral friend Beaumont called them. Smoking a Pall Mall in a tiny Triumph was like smoking in a one-man elevator, but we didn't give a rip. When the smoke got so thick our eyes burned, we took a break and rolled down the windows.

"Cigarette smoke keeps the mosquitoes away," proclaimed Brainy Beau that night, and who was I to question a genius? After saying that, and while making tracks up my thigh highway, he jerked back and slapped at a mosquito the size of a bat. It flew out the window with a chunk of Beau's left cheek.

"Time for another ciggie, babe," he mumbled, and down came the windows. We stopped huffing and started puffing. Our Pall Malls were non-filtered, so every now and then, Beaumont spit a piece of tobacco out of the side of his mouth using his tongue. I didn't spit mine out. When I felt that hard little grain of tobacco, I swished it around until it was on the tip of my tongue. Very carefully, I lifted it with my thumb and forefinger and flicked it out of the open window like Brenda Starr might have done.

When the Spitfire got smoked up again and looked more like a hookah bar than the inside of a sports car, we threw away the butts, rolled the windows back up and Beaumont resumed thumb-circling my thigh. He didn't start at my knee, and he didn't kiss me either. I wanted him to, because

I envisioned Beaumont, the Spitfire and Moi all exploding like cherry bombs on the Fourth of July. That's how the bodice rippers always depicted the big number.

Beaumont must have read my thoughts because he took his left hand, pulled my right shoulder toward him and began to lick my lips like a cat taking a bath. Then he stuck his tongue slightly into my mouth and ran it slowly across my front teeth.

Now, if you had told me the day before that this was called "foreplay" and something I should expect, I'd have said nobody was going to lick my teeth. But when it happened, I figured tongue-to-teeth kissing was another experience I would write about someday.

Ol' Beaumont was a good kisser. By the time he got around to the long, wet French kiss I had learned about before I could drive a car, I was another Lady Chatterley.

So caught up was I in that tongue of his that I scarcely noticed his hands groping under my sweater. By the time I felt the awkward jerk of my bra clasp, I wasn't sure if Beaumont's fingers had loosened it or if my inner heat had popped it open like a jack-in-the-box.

His hands found both of my bee-sting boobies and within seconds, he got busy doing loop-the-loops. It was feeling pretty good until the fool pinched one of my sweet virginal nips.

"Ouch!" I yelled.

Beaumont jumped like he'd been cow-prodded, but then quickly moved on to greener pastures. He lifted my sweater as he took his lips away from my mouth, lowered his head and almost apologetically kissed my tiny pinched-up breast.

I don't know how he managed to do it, but before I could say, "Whoa, cowboy," Beaumont had crawled over the gearshift and the parking brake and was on his knees in front of me in a space barely big enough for a Shih Tzu. He gently pushed up my gored skirt and began rotating his thumb south.

Breathing heavily, he mumbled, "You still a virgin?"

It was now or never. Sink or swim. It was the eleventh hour. I could back out and never risk being called a hussy. Or I could . . .

"Get cracking, Beau. I ain't getting no younger."

The next day, I took off all of my clothes and stood in front of the floor-length mirror in my bedroom. I thought if I stared at myself long enough, I would see a different girl from the one that had left the house in a wide, gored skirt the night before.

I thought my drab dishwater blonde hair might have turned into a blaze of crimson, a la Brenda Starr. That my eyes, now filled with carnal knowledge, would have turned into blue, sparkling stars like hers, and that my facial expression would broadcast the fact that I was now a card-carrying, full-fledged woman.

I waited there in front of the mirror for a long time, gazing at myself, hopeful as only the young can be. No discernable difference became apparent. I would have to live for many more years before learning that awakenings, like clouds, can be full, puffy and distinguishable. More often, however, they are just full of hot air.

# Wanna Do It?

by
Laura Steidl

Our 10 years of married life were good, but often mundane. You could say my husband and I were in a marital rut, and I was hungry for something different to break up the monotony.

Sometimes I thought about the old cliché, "Variety is the spice of life," and wondered if boredom was what drove married people into having affairs. Did they intentionally go looking for someone different, or did it just happen? I had been wondering if I needed to have an affair to spice up my life.

Burrowed deep under the covers of our double bed and contemplating the complications of divorce and an affair outside of marriage, I heard my husband come home from work. After working from 3 P.M. to 11 P.M., he liked to drink a beer and read the newspaper—undisturbed by conversation with me—before going to bed. That was the reason I hadn't stayed up to greet him. Comforted by knowing he was home, I drifted off to sleep.

Later, I awoke when the floorboards creaked in protest as my husband walked around our bedroom in the dark. I heard a faint *click* when he placed his watch on the dresser. His belt buckle jingled softly as he pulled his legs out of his blue jeans. My mind formed pictures in my head of his bare masculine body while rustling noises whispered to me that he was removing the rest of his clothes. When he was naked, he lifted the covers on his side of the bed and carefully slipped between the sheets, slowly inching his way in my direction until I felt the warmth of his body next to mine.

Then I faintly heard, "Wanna do it?" Experience had taught me that question meant having a sexual quickie without foreplay, with his only interest in his climatic pleasure, not mine.

I craved some pleasuring too, so I ignored his request for effortless sex and feigned being asleep. After a few minutes of silence, his hand reached up and rubbed my neck. It felt good and I liked it. Soon he was gently licking and sucking on the back of my shoulder. I liked that, too.

"Hi, baby. Daddy's home. Why don't you roll over? I can't rub all of your good parts when you're lying on your stomach."

His efforts of foreplay deserved reward, so I faked stirring out of my pretend sleep and rolled onto my back. We exchanged a long wet kiss as he pressed his hard manhood against my thigh. I soon became titillated. When he fumbled with my nightgown to unveil my breasts, I helped him by sitting up and raising my arms so he could pull it off over my head.

I swear guys have six hands, and his were all over me. But I didn't mind. While he touched and rubbed me, I stroked and rubbed him in all his favorite places. He knew where I liked to be touched and exactly how much pressure to apply. Too rough and I complain. Too light and it tickles so much I scream and holler. That happened a few times during our first month of marriage, and he never made that mistake again. He thought he was in bed with a banshee, and it proved to be a real mood breaker. Knowing what your partner likes is a big advantage not available with a stranger.

It didn't take long before the kissing, hugging, sucking and rubbing we were doing to each other made our heavy breathing get pretty loud. I think we could have rivaled a freight train! Suddenly, I started to worry that our kids might wake up and hear us having sex. Our nine-year-old had a bedroom next to ours and his 10-year-old brother was across the hall. All the bedroom doors were open.

"We have to stop! We can't wake the kids!" I said.

But he refused to quit, not at the point we were just about to do it! He begged and pleaded with me to continue, but I was certain our kids would hear us. Plus, my amorous mood had faded.

"Honey, please don't take it personal. I love you. I really do want to make love with you. I just don't want the kids to hear us. Please try to understand." Then I began to cry. My tears always melted his heart.

In a sympathetic voice, he asked, "What if we go some-place where the kids can't hear us?"

"Where can we go? They'll hear us in the house, and we can't leave them home alone."

"We don't have to leave home. Let's go outside and do it in the car."

I stopped crying and thought about how we used to park the car in secret hide-a-way places to have sex before we were married. The idea sounded naughty and exciting.

"OK," I said.

I grabbed the quilt off the bed, wrapped it around my naked body and followed my husband outside. Shameless, he walked out the door naked. I didn't see any houses with lights on as we quietly sneaked barefoot across the black-topped driveway to the car. A big poplar tree shaded the car from the city streetlights. After we had got in, we carefully closed the doors so as not to make any noise. I didn't want neighbors getting startled and calling the police. And I didn't want them watching us, either.

Lilac bushes kept the car from being seen by the neighbors who lived on the lot behind us. I was satisfied we now had the privacy I needed to feel comfortable about what we intended to do. It helped that our street was always quiet, especially late at night. The sky glowed softly from a beautiful display of bright stars that seemed to be shining just for me, and the waxing crescent moon looked like a crooked smile. The temperature had dropped to a cool 62 degrees, making us both glad I had brought the quilt.

Now that my fear of waking the kids was gone, our passion quickly returned, and we were able to consummate our lovemaking in the safety of our car. In the house, fear of discovery was debilitating. In the car, fear of discovery added to the excitement!

After that, my husband and I often had sex in the car under the cover of darkness. It was fun and made me feel like a newlywed again. The car's shape and limited space required experimenting with new, and sometimes twisted, positions. We discovered a new meaning for the word "variety," especially when spicing up our marriage and our love life.

# The U-Turn

by
### Nick E. Lodeon

College is one of those times when you do stupid things for stupid reasons—or for no reason other than trying to save a few bucks.

For me, money was always on the short side, so being frugal was something I and a few of my friends practiced. Like the time a bunch of us guys decided to scale the fence into the horse races rather than pay a few measly bucks at the gate. Trouble was, someone who likely paid the $2 entry fee reported five guys scrambling over the fence. Five minutes after we sat down in the stands, the cops showed up and escorted us out. We did pay to get back in legally, but missed the first race.

One of my friends drove a Ford Galaxy, back in the days when gas cost 40-cents per gallon. Great thing about his car was that it had a humongous trunk and drive-in movies were still quite popular. So climbing into the trunk to save money was a given. Usually it wasn't an issue jumping in there, and in fact three or four of us often argued about who sat in the passenger seats and got stuck paying to get in. But the night John and I decided to take our girlfriends to the drive-in created some trepidation about asking either of the girls to climb into the trunk. Fortunately, the girl I'd been dating for a month was a free-loving hippie and was game to try anything crazy.

"Why don't you and I climb in the trunk and sneak in?" Kat asked. "That way we've got more money for beer."

I laughed. "Are you sure? Gets dark in there."

"You aren't afraid of the dark, are you?" she teased.

"It gets hot, too," I added.

"Promise?" she said, smiling that quirky smile of hers. She started unbuttoning her blouse, but stopped once she got far enough for me to see that her large, perky breasts had no bothersome bra supporting them. Who was I to argue?

All four of us initially climbed into the car's passenger seats as we headed for the drive-in. When we stopped at a small market to purchase our required cheap wine, beer and food supply, Kat and I announced our trunk intentions. It was already dark when Kat and I crawled into the trunk and she quickly unbuttoned her blouse all the way.

"Take your time getting there, John," I said as he closed the trunk. As I settled into those beauties, John and his girl-friend climbed back into the front seat, and off we went. It got really hot in a hurry in that trunk. After about 10 minutes of driving, on a trip that should have taken only five minutes to get there, we heard John yell, "I missed the turn-off!"

"Great!" I yelled back—more time for Kat and me to spend alone. I headed back to work, but stopped when Kat and I felt the car suddenly speed up.

"Aren't we going kind of fast?" Kat asked, sounding a bit concerned.

"Hey, John, what the hell are you doing?!" I yelled through the backseat from inside the trunk.

There was no answer. The car simply went faster.

"John, damn it. What the hell are you doing?"

"We're on the freeway," he yelled back.

"Freeway? What the hell are you doing on the freeway?!"

There was no answer. Suddenly, the car slowed then made a hard left turn, bounced over some really rough roadway, made another hard left turn back onto a smooth roadway and accelerated again.

"John, what the hell are you doing?! Where are you going?!" I yelled again.

Kat grabbed me around my ass and squeezed, pulling me closer to her, which was quite a feat considering how close we already were. "Are we going to die?" she asked, only half-joking.

"No, but John may not live after we get out of here," I said, also only half joking.

Another turn and we finally slowed to a more reasonable speed. Then there was a quick little turn to the right and we were back on rough terrain.

"John, are we at the drive-in yet?!"

"No, a cop is pulling me over!" he yelled back. "Shut up and don't say anything!"

Kat giggled. "This is getting pretty exciting."

"I'm not sure 'exciting' is how I would describe this," I said, now worried.

We heard the car's door open and slam closed, and then someone—I assumed John—walking through gravel alongside the trunk. There was a light tap-tap on the trunk. "Quiet you two," John said in a loud whisper. "The cop is getting out of his car."

Kat and I lay there, her bare breasts heaving up and down as her breathing increased.

Suddenly, without any warning, the trunk popped open and its light came on. All Kat and I saw was a bright flashlight beam aimed at us as we both struggled to sit up. The light dropped a bit and we saw that the startled cop had drawn his gun and was aiming it directly at us.

"Don't shoot! We're just sneaking into the drive-in!" I yelled. I looked at Kat and all I saw was her 38D's pointing at the cop's .38, and his startled look slowly turning into a giant smile as he realized her 38D's would do him no harm. I quickly pulled my pants back up.

The cop started laughing. We started laughing, although ours was more of a nervous laugh. He told Kat and I to get out of the trunk. He then gave John a ticket for making an illegal U-turn on the freeway, over the median; then he kicked us loose.

We watched as the cop returned to his patrol car. As

soon as he pulled away, I turned to John. "Why did you open the trunk?" I asked him.

"Uh," he babbled, "Ahh, I thought maybe he would hear you two breathing or laughing and maybe he'd start shooting at the trunk."

"Bullshit, that's bullshit. Don't ever do that again, please," I said. I grabbed Kat's hand and we climbed back into the trunk.

"What are you doing?" John asked.

"We're getting back into the trunk because we spent all our money on beer." I hesitated, studying John's face for a moment. "We *are* still going to the movies, aren't we?"

"Uh, yeah, I guess." He looked at his girlfriend, who hadn't moved from her position in the front seat. With more determination, he said, "Of course we're still going to the drive-in. I need to get something for what's likely to be a $50 ticket."

John closed the trunk on Kat and me, and this time, he didn't miss the turn-off into the drive-in.

# A Long and Winding Road

by
Dierdre Jackson

My husband's business trips could be called anything but interesting to me. In the early years of our marriage, I had accompanied him on several, simply because I hated to spend evenings alone. Rare, overnight trips proved more interesting. We could not afford a honeymoon after we got married, so we called an occasional night in a motel a "mini-honeymoon." I learned that Champagne and silk sheets were not necessary to insure a night filled with spine-tingling kisses and great sex with my guy.

After we had two children in three years, my husband changed jobs. The business trips ceased. Eventually, he formed his own company, which again necessitated overnight trips to see new clients. I no longer minded staying at home when he had to be gone. I even welcomed an occasional evening alone. After the children were finished with homework and baths then safely tucked into bed, I could read as long as I chose.

Time passed, and I found myself the mother of two teenagers—one 16, the other, 18. When my husband announced he had an upcoming trip through the Ozarks, it held a certain appeal. We lived in Central Missouri at the time, and I had often thought that it might be nice to vacation in the Ozarks. But the time had never been right for us to do so.

"When is it?" I asked.

"I need to leave next Thursday. I have a meeting in Poplar Bluff at 3 P.M., which will take at least two hours, maybe three. Then I'll drive to West Plains, find a motel and meet with the second guy at nine the next morning."

I thought about it for a few minutes before I spoke. "Is there any reason I can't go with you? The kids will be fine. I could ask the neighbors to keep an eye out for them."

He seemed surprised. "Well, sure. I thought you didn't like my boring meetings." He grinned, the lop-sided grin I had found so appealing when we were teenagers.

"The trees should be beautiful down there right now." I reminded him that it was, after all, the middle of October, and a near-full moon would soon be upon us.

He wiggled his eyebrows. "It's a date!" He seemed eager at the thought.

Thursday morning, six days later, with my overnight bag packed with a change of clothing and new lingerie (just in case) and an instruction list on the kitchen table for the kids, I climbed into the passenger seat of our 1977 two-door Bonneville, ready for whatever magic I could whip up overnight. The day could not have been more perfect. Not a single cloud marred the October-blue sky, the shade of blue that always stirred something inside my heart, perhaps a latent call of the wild.

We left right after the children went to school, not wanting to be rushed on the four-hour drive south to Poplar Bluff. We stopped for a leisurely lunch in a local diner along the way, chatting and enjoying our time together.

A good, thick paperback book in my hands, I was satisfied to sit in the outer office of the building where his first appointment took place. Occasionally, I glanced at my watch, in no hurry, but conscious that dusk fell quickly at that time of year.

At 5:30, my husband and his client came from the inner office, shook hands and we left. "I told Mr. Sherman that we were driving to West Plains to spend the night, so he called information to see if there is a motel." (Back then, there were no cellphones or GPS, but only, "Information, please.")

"I hope there's at least one," I said. I had unhappy visions of an ugly "no-tell-motel" at the side of a country road.

"There is exactly one," he said. "And we got the last room in it!"

I wondered if my thoughts of a soft, wide bed in a room far away from vending and ice machines would be an unfulfilled dream.

"Oh, well, the map shows that it's only 70 or 80 miles. Let's get something to eat here. I'm hungry," my husband suggested.

By the time we left the restaurant, the last glimmer of

sunset swiftly faded away. My husband pointed the car west, and we soon discovered that the two-lane highway held successions of curves—practically switchbacks—with speed limits of 25 mph to 35 mph posted at every one.

My husband hated curvy roads. The inside of our car grew very quiet. Dense woods lined both sides of the road. We were unable to tell how extensive they were, but I noticed that not many houses were visible. Aside from a few rundown farmhouses and rusty trailers, civilization seemed somewhat scarce.

Then the most beautiful moon I had ever seen cast a glow so bright that we scarcely needed headlights to see the road. I found a country music station on the radio, and there was Patsy Cline crooning *Crazy*. I hummed along with her, harmonizing.

I scooted closer to my husband on the car's bench seat and placed my hand on his thigh.

"Careful there, girlie," he said, chuckling. "Don't start somethin' you don't mean to finish."

"I'm not."

He slowed the car to accommodate the impending 30 mph curve. "Have you noticed that there is no traffic on this road?"

"Yes." I snuggled underneath his right shoulder, just as I had done 20 years earlier. "I've seen what looks like several little trails into the woods, but no houses."

He didn't answer me, but I continued to trail my hand along his thigh, careful not to distract him completely. I had no desire for the car to end up against a tree.

From the radio, Ronnie Milsap's velvet voice pleaded

*Please Don't Tell Me How the Story Ends*. The car slowed and stopped. My husband then carefully backed into a barely visible lane. Trees formed a barrier on all sides and blocked us from the highway, should anyone drive by.

"Can you still climb over the seat? " he asked, motioning to the back. I could hear the hopeful teasing in his voice.

"Just watch me." I was 38 years old, not quite as svelte as I had been the last time I had done such a thing, but I accomplished the challenge quite easily.

He started to follow me. "Dang!"

"What's wrong?" A moment of absolute panic swept over me, afraid that we had been discovered.

"My pants pocket caught on the gear shift!"

I laughed, and suddenly there he was, right beside me.

It didn't take us long to work out the logistics of an unfamiliar backseat, laughing all the way, until we were no longer laughing. I completely forgot about the silky, black lingerie in my bag. I forgot about everything except the handsome, exciting, familiar man who held me with passion and tenderness, as he had for over two decades.

What I discovered that night, somewhere between Poplar Bluff and West Plains, Missouri, was what it does not take to experience good sex. It does not take Champagne, silk sheets, a wide bed in an expensive room, teasing lingerie, the perfect setting or any of the other trappings. It takes two people who love each other.

Of course, a full moon on an October night, hidden away on a country lane, in the backseat of a paid-for-car doesn't hurt, either.

# From Midget to Mammoth

by
## Samantha Johnson

"Off! Get off! Get off NOW! It isn't meant to bend like this," Steve whimpered like a puppy.

I thought his moaning indicated he'd been enjoying himself and was about to climax. Um, obviously not. Attempting to relieve his pain, I had difficulty moving off him because the steering wheel was buried into my spine. To make matters worse, my knee slipped between the car seat and the car door. I slammed back down with my entire weight at an even more uncomfortable angle. The only choice I had was to open the car door and literally slide off a quickly vanishing erection and right onto the ground.

"Gee, that was fun, huh?" I stifled a giggle as I stood up.

My tough, rugged lover wiped sweat from his forehead.

"Why would anyone in their right mind drive an M.G. Midget?" I then asked. "You've got to trade cars or something before one of us is seriously injured."

We were both tall, and to maneuver about in Steve's car was damn-near impossible. And believe me, we tried every conceivable position known to man. Penetration ranged from difficult to impossible—unless you count the gearshift up my ass a few times.

Our relationship was wonderful but overloaded with obstacles from day one. We worked full time, lived 40 miles apart and still resided with our parents. We had little time for dating, let alone romance in that tiny auto. And as for privacy—we had zilch.

Yearning for long, drawn out, passionate sex, I finally had a light-bulb moment and wondered why it had taken me so long. Big Daddy's pastures! I don't recall ever calling my father by any other name, nor do I know where I picked up that one.

My family raised cattle, and we had numerous pastures with locks on the gates. Guess who knew all the combinations? Talk about privacy—Steve and I would have it made in rural Oklahoma.

Sure, the Midget was still an issue until we finally resorted to keeping a blanket behind the seat. With it spread out on lush, grassy pastureland, we escaped into nirvana with no aches, pains or bruises. And that's when we realized we weren't just in lust; we were in love. The only thing we had to fear in our secret hide-a-way was a stampede of cattle should coyotes be lurking about.

After an unusually late romp in the pasture one evening, when I got home, I took a quick shower and dove into bed, hoping sleep would come quickly. I worked the next day and was exhausted.

The following day went well until right after lunch. Then the itching began! I wandered in and out of empty offices and conference rooms so I could reach my crotch and butt. Scratching and rubbing only intensified my problem. *Chiggers, it has to be chiggers*, I thought.

Going out of my mind, I eventually ducked into the bathroom to scrutinize the situation. "Crap," I gasped. I didn't find one chigger, but instead, found an acute case of poison ivy. No doubt, it had happened when I'd squatted behind some bushes before heading home the evening before. It had been a pitch-black night, and I had assumed it was prairie grass tickling my girlie parts while I peed like a racehorse. Wrong!

Fibbing, I told my boss I had a prescription waiting for me at the pharmacy about a block away, and I casually left the building. When I got to the pharmacy, I had a private consultation with the pharmacist, and then watched him bag up a blue bottle that looked familiar.

While he fiddled with the cash register making change, I peeked inside the bag. *Milk Of Magnesia?!* I shoved the bottle toward him. "Are you serious? I didn't say I was constipated, I have poison ivy! I don't need diarrhea, too."

He had the nerve to smile, "It's one of the best cures around, but few people know it. People have used it for generations. Just trust me, or wait until you can see your doctor. It's your choice."

Brown bag in hand, I hustled back to work, hid in a

bathroom stall and slathered on the milky liquid. While applying the so-called cure-all, I rubbed my fingers over a bump that startled me. Something wasn't right. *A blister that large from poison ivy? No way.*

I yanked a mirror from my purse to investigate more closely. *What the hell?!* Closer examination revealed the largest tick I'd ever seen. It was so gorged with blood, I feared it might explode any minute! Being a country gal, I'd had many of those blasted bugs attach themselves to me, but this one was gargantuan. There's an art to tick removal—and my personal assistant had always been Big Daddy. Well, I was on my own this time since the tick was affixed to my twat.

Exiting the ladies' room, I casually approached a co-worker who smoked and asked for a cigarette. "Samantha, you don't smoke!" Donna said, shocked.

"Um, no I don't. But it's the only remedy I know of for tick removal unless you have a better one." She handed me a cig promptly, along with a book of matches.

"I don't want you to burn yourself. I'll come help if it's in a hard-to-reach location," she offered.

"No problem, I've got it. Thanks."

Inside the stall, I spread my legs, lit the cigarette and bent from the waist like a contortionist. Carefully, very carefully, I singed the rear of the tick then waited a few seconds. That sucker was still holding on! During the procedure, I singed a few pubic hairs, as well. The bathroom reeked with the stench. *Nice.*

Before my next attempt, I spit on my fingers first to tame any wild hairs. Then I let that disgusting bug have it until my delicate, female tissue was all but scorched. "Whoo hoo and hot damn!" I said chuckling aloud when that blood sucker finally dropped to the floor. For good measure, I stomped on it, too.

When I shared my day with Steve, he laughed hearing about the condition my private parts were in. I wanted to kick him. What with the weather turning cold soon, the only option we now had was celibacy, at least until spring. His car was too small, and we couldn't even afford a cheap, ratty motel room. And after reading up on poison ivy, we weren't having sex for several more weeks, anyway.

Within days, Steve proposed to me and we opted for a run-away wedding. It was planned for exactly the time I'd be healed from the poison ivy. On our wedding night, what joy it was to have sex in a bed for the first time ever! The shower was especially romantic as we lathered up, tantalizing one another under the running water, later on the kitchen table, and then the recliner. The list goes on, and we tried everything—we couldn't get enough of each other.

But then, four kids and 10 years later, we found ourselves right back where we began. Our desire for sex had not diminished, but we had four sets of peering eyes and little ears. Again our privacy was zilch. Kudos to the company that invented RVs. Ours, which is big enough to park three M.G. Midgets inside, includes a high-tech monitor to keep tabs on the kids in the house, and it's parked just steps away from the backdoor. Yes, size does matter.

# What's the Expiration Date of Sex?

There is none!

# Games People Play

by
Marlene Cloude

Party games. By the time you're looking at your golden years, if you've played one, you've played them all. I needed to come up with a new and exciting game for a bunch of older lady friends to play at the annual Bag Lady picnic.

I searched the Internet high and low for something other than Bingo or word scrambles. So boring. Then I stumbled onto a site that listed "Handbag Scavenger Hunt," and I realized the possibilities were endless. My invitations went out, instructing the gals to come prepared the day of the picnic with everything but the kitchen sink in their handbags.

Then I began to brainstorm the many items I would call out for the ladies to extract from their bags during the picnic. Each item on the list was assigned a random point value. Those things that most people would carry were given a low number. The more difficult items had a higher point value.

There would be a special prize for the winner.

First, I listed the usual and expected items—cellphone, keys, makeup, pill box, tissue, sunglasses, wallet, pictures of grandchildren, candy, breath mints and pens. Then, I listed more that might not usually be carried—flashlight, tape measure, CD, screwdriver, hairnet, camera, apple, recent grocery receipt, gloves, jewelry, scissors, sewing kit, hair salon appointment card, fan, discount card, book, church bulletin and others.

Finally, the website suggested that the highly unusual and unexpected addition of a condom as the final item would add a new dimension and fun to the activity. I loved the idea! The condom was to be "planted" with the person in the group that everyone would least expect to have it.

But there was one hitch: I needed to plant something else other than a condom, just in case I wasn't the only one in the group who was familiar with this game. That's when I remembered a past shopping trip for a bachelorette party. I had come upon cherry-flavored edible underwear. *That's it!* I thought. Even though this was a fun-loving group, I didn't think even one of my guests would think to put edible undies in her handbag on the off chance they would be needed for the game. I envisioned initial shock, laughter, gasps and catcalls when I would call out that last item.

My husband accompanied me on a trip to the mall to purchase the underwear. I admit I was a little uncomfortable. When I asked where to find the item, a female salesclerk said the panties were located toward the back of the store. That meant far away from the jewelry, Gothic-looking items, psychedelic posters and lava lamps. Further, the sexual-oriented stock was kept behind a curtain with a sign above the entrance that read, "Must Be 18 Years Old to Enter."

Worried we might run into friends while we shopped in the sex department, I stressed even more when I noticed that my husband was eagerly looking at all the other things he envisioned would spice up our bedroom life!

"Hey. Look at this! It's a vibrator that goes on the end of my tongue!" he said loudly as he winked at me suggestively. "And look at this thing! It has two vibrating heads! How do you think it's supposed to work?"

Seriously? Did he really expect me to explain it to him?

I left him turning the two-headed dildo over and over in his hands while I continued to look for the panties. As I turned the corner and found what I had come for, I heard a continuous buzz behind me—my husband had found the ON switch for the toy he was fondling. I grabbed the undies and hurried my husband toward the checkout counter—without the dildo—but not before he made one more attempt to talk me into the tongue vibrator.

"Forget it! For $5.99, all that thing is going to do is make you stutter, vibrate your false teeth out of your head and loosen your fillings, to boot!" I said. He was disappointed to leave without it, but we both laughed as we made our way to the front of the store picturing that intimate bedroom fiasco.

Stepping up to the counter to pay for my prized cherry-flavored edible panties, the register clerk turned around. My face flamed, my eyes grew round and my heart rate increased tenfold. I had forgotten that the very handsome young son of good family friends managed the store. He smiled broadly as he acknowledged us both.

"Did you find everything that you came in for?" he asked. I rolled my eyes. *Could this get any worse?*

"Oh, she sure did," said my husband as he turned and walked away, his shoulders convulsed with suppressed laughter.

I took a deep breath and calmly put the edible undies on the counter as I reached for my wallet. To his credit, the handsome friend-of-the-family never blinked, and his face never changed as he rang up my purchase, took my money and placed the undies in a bag. But it was too much for me. I felt the need to explain.

"These are not for us! I am hosting a picnic this weekend, and they're a gag gift for a prize," I said. "Please don't mention this to your parents. We will never hear the end of it." He just smiled and gave me my sack.

The weather was perfect, and the turnout for our picnic couldn't have been better. Many of the attendees carried oversized handbags in anticipation of the scavenger hunt. We all laughed as the many items on the list were called out and were eagerly produced for all to see.

"Ladies, we have one final item. If you have this item in your bag, it's worth 50 points!" I said. Guests looked at each other quizzically, wondering what could possibly illicit such a high point value. I paused dramatically so everyone would hear my request clearly.

"Has anyone brought a pair of cherry-flavored edible underwear in her handbag?" I asked. Just as I expected, the pavilion instantly erupted with sounds of laughter as ladies teased each other about the final item.

Suddenly, from the back of the pavilion, a small, elderly, stooped woman who walked with a cane stood and shouted gleefully, "I think I have that in my handbag!" More laughter and shouting ensued as I invited her to bring her bag to the front and produce the tasty garment.

Sure enough, she pulled out a pair of cherry-flavored edible undies as the other ladies clapped, hollered and cheered for her! Her award for accruing the most points was a tongue vibrator that was purchased by my husband. He suggested it was the perfect prize since it came described as "A great addition to your handbag and your next weekend trip. The small size of this vibrator sex toy makes it a fantastic way to surprise your lover!" Not to mention all your pals who think fun, games and sex ends at 80!

# Cobwebs on the Ceiling

by
Kathy Whirity

I was 23 years old and newly married when my husband, Bill, and I moved into our first home. The minute we got out of the car, we were introduced to our new neighbor. To us, she seemed like an old lady, though looking back, she was probably in her early 50s, much younger than I am now.

The first thing she said to us was that we would have to take better care of our lawn than the previous owners did.

We mumbled, "Nice to meet you, too," as we hurried into the house.

We met her husband the night he came home drunk, fell to the ground and couldn't get up. I watched out our front window on that cold January night as he lay there, trying to stand. He kept moving his legs, which caused him to spin in a circle, going nowhere on the icy sidewalk.

It didn't take us long to figure out that she was the Nosy Rosy of the neighborhood, and he was an abusive husband when he drank—which was almost every night.

One summer evening, my husband and I heard them yelling and fighting. There was no denying he was drunk—his foul language was a dead giveaway. Our back porch windows were in proximity to their bedroom, so we crouched beneath one of the windows and listened. We had, at times, done this out of concern for her. In the short time we had lived there, the police had frequently been called to intervene.

We listened closely, our ears pressed close to the window screen. There was no mistaking what he was ranting and raving about—he wanted to have sex, and she was apparently ignoring his advances.

Holding our hands over our mouths, we couldn't help but stifle a laugh. At our age, it was hilarious to us that two gray-haired "older" folks would still be having sex at all. The old man yelled at Nosy Rosy and was overly obnoxious about wanting her to come to bed—RIGHT NOW!

Then, all of a sudden, there was dead silence. We looked at each other and guessed he had passed out. At least we hoped so, for her sake.

As we stood up to close the patio windows, the silence was broken by Mr. Rosy yelling as loud as he could, "There are cobwebs on the ceiling! How do you expect me to $%&# with cobwebs on the ceiling?!" We began laughing so hard; we had to run into the kitchen, only sneaking onto the back porch much later to close the opened windows.

My husband and I tried to guess what had happened in their bedroom. Did the wife have a change of heart and decide to please her man? We imagined her walking to bed, willing to do the deed and mount her man, only to be admonished for bad housekeeping. It was the one and only time we ever heard him be so vocal about lovemaking—or lack thereof.

I laugh whenever I think about the night that cobwebs on the ceiling thwarted their sexcapades. No wonder the husband's instances of getting lucky were so rare. And I learned something from our eavesdropping that long ago night: Yes, old people do have sex!

# Vaginaplasty

by
Georgia Mellie Justad

You've got to be kidding!

I could hardly believe my ears as the overly enthusiastic woman chattered away on the radio, advertising the latest "two-fer special" to sweep Boca Raton. It was for, of all things, a vaginaplasty.

"Direct from Beverly Hills, this popular surgical procedure is now available in South Florida. And for a limited time, you can bring a friend during this Super Summertime Special. Yes, ladies, who wants to walk around with a droopy vagina when you can have a perkier, tighter one?"

I tried to imagine the conversation that would take place when I called my BFF to pitch the idea of spending the afternoon having our vaginas lifted or perked up or whatever they do. "Hey, girlfriend, what are you doing next Saturday? They've got a special at our local plastic surgery salon. Something that will perk us right up." Well, I did just that, and I giggled as she howled at the idea. Needless to say, she passed.

And perky? What's up with that? Who knows what makes a vagina droopy? It could be depressed, in a bad mood or maybe in need of a little vacation after years of service. Or maybe it requires therapy to perk it up. There's a person for that—a vaginal motivational speaker. I think Boca Raton can corner the market on that one. We have everything else: the horse whisperer, the dog whisperer, so why not the vagina whisperer? It could be a natural alternative to surgery. And who wouldn't want that—a happy, well-adjusted, carefree vagina? I can imagine the vaginal motivational speaker saying from the stage to hundreds of downtrodden vaginas, "Hello down there, little vaginas. How are you all today? You're certainly looking well."

I had no clue what a vaginaplasty would entail and what type of desperate woman would consider the procedure. After some research, I discovered that a vaginaplasty—or "vaginal rejuvenation"—is primarily for older women who want to tighten up their aging (and apparently decrepit) vaginas, restoring them to their youthful, pre-pregnancy days. Well, who wouldn't want that? I don't know how I every made it to the age of 50 without the surgery, but obviously, I was now the prime age for it.

To be honest, I wasn't quite sure if my vagina was droopy or not. But since everything else on my body had been going south as of late, maybe I wasn't as safe as I'd initially thought. At least my vagina hadn't made it past my now slightly sagging, circus-elephant knees.

When it came to the commercial announcer mentioning

a "tighter" vagina, whose idea was that? I imagine this male-inspired procedure was an entirely new way for a woman to "get a grip" and return to her days of "hands-free" pole dancing. I ask you, what woman cares if her vagina has gone a little loosey-goosey over time, as long as it's not sitting in the crotch of her panties?

I have no problem with plastic surgery to tweak a little here and there, but hell, half the fun of having work done is letting everybody get a good look at the new and improved you afterward. So how do you debut your new vagina during your "coming out" luncheon? Crotchless panties would be a bit too tasteless. Maybe I could do a few cheesy, under-the-table parlor tricks to impress my friends, like dropping a spoon on the floor and deftly sucking it up, hands-free, without so as a much as a sweat.

"I don't see anything wrong with it," Hubby said—just like a man—when I told him about the ludicrous procedure I had heard advertised on the radio.

Poor Hubby. Since my hysterectomy, I'd banished him to the guest room, my hot flashes and night sweats more than I could handle. He had been reduced to scratching at my bedroom door for the occasional conjugal visit.

A few months later, with the preposterous vaginaplasty idea gone from my mind and a full recovery from my hysterectomy, Hubby and I were once again doing the "dance with no pants." Let me tell you, peeing when you sneeze isn't the worst thing that can happen while performing your wifely duties. In the middle of our fun, right before climax, I unexpectedly sneezed and . . . how do I put this delicately . . . well, there isn't really a way . . . I . . . uh . . . "spit him out," if you catch my drift.

Yep. It. Out.

"What the hell?!" he asked, deflating as I giggled. I popped another estrogen pill as if it were a Skittle.

"The doctor never told me that *this* could happen," I said, matter of factly, as I scanned over the "What to Expect After Your Hysterectomy" info packet.

"Your menopause has ruined my life!" my long-suffering hubby exclaimed, putting his new sexy silk underwear—a waste of money, of course—back on.

"Oh, my God. You're kidding me!" my BFF exploded as I recounted my boudoir bedlam. "You didn't! That's hilarious! What did he do?"

"The whole thing took him by surprise, as if he'd been thrown from a horse. He looked insulted, and then rejected, as if I had done it on purpose. You know, like he had given me a present and I had thrown it back at him."

"It would appear you did," she said, laughing.

"He's still pouting, bless his heart. In the meantime, I'm trying to make sure it doesn't happen again. I've brushed up on my Kegel exercises, and I've got a bottle of Claritin D on my nightstand."

Not long after, I visited the gynecologist and was met with a speech about how once you hit 50, your hormones are depleted.

"Your vagina goes downhill," the doctor continued, in her all-knowing 35-year-old voice. With my feet in those horrible stirrups, she peered at my lady parts. Her tone sounded as if she was personally going to put my va-jay-jay out to pasture right then and there.

"Sounds like you're suggesting I shoot for early retirement," I said, wishing the entire humiliating examination would be over quickly.

"My, would you look at this!" the doctor then said excitedly, her speculum still in place.

*What now?* I thought to myself. *Did she discover the Loch Ness monster hiding there?*

"Your hormone replacement and Kegel exercises are certainly paying off. Yes, indeedy. Your vagina looks healthy, firm and fresh," she gushed.

Yep, that's the word she used—fresh. Like a loaf of Wonder Bread.

"Have a look for yourself," she said.

*Have a look? How? I'm not a contortionist!*

"Over here," she said, spinning a huge monitor by my head.

Frankly, never having seen *it*, I didn't recognize *it* at first. I was flabbergasted as I came face to face with *it* for the first time. I imagined an announcer saying, "Brought to you in living color and HD cinema scope—it's your vagina!" Was I a medical miracle or a porn star? I wasn't sure.

"You know," the doctor commented, still clearly impressed. "You have the vagina of a 25-year-old."

I looked at her in disbelief. *I'll be damned.*

Thanking her for the compliment, I said, "Been a long time since I've heard that! I suppose that means no vaginaplasty for me." Wouldn't you know it? I was able to turn back the evil hands of time, and I couldn't even show it off.

I left the doctor's office, my head high, knowing that at least part of me was younger than half the women in the waiting room. There's nothing quite like taking 25 years off the old "vaginal" clock. Just don't tell Hubby. He doesn't need any more encouragement!

# Normal, Normal, Normal

by
Phyllis G. Westover

"Normal, normal, normal," my husband always says while checking the gauges of our second 1991 Ford Explorer, the one he's been cheering on to 200,000 miles. Sure enough, the temperature, oil and battery needles all pointed in the normal charging zones.

Our trips to Colorado necessitate a car that's trustworthy. We bought Explorer Two third-hand after a freak accident totaled beloved Explorer One. With its odometer pushing 160,000 miles, Explorer Two has had its repairs and parts replacements: a new radiator, a new serpentine belt to replace the one that snapped just before we climbed Wolf Creek Pass and new brake disks and pads before descending from Breckenridge. We travel with books to read aloud, favorite CDs and a bottle of steering fluid between our front seats to replenish the chronic leak we've yet to fix.

Such maintenance sets me thinking about our condition—

we who didn't meet until we were over half a century old, each having a second go at marriage after first ones broke down. We, too, have had our repairs and replacements: a hip replacement and rotor-rooter job for my husband, and a hip and knee replacement for me, plus saying adios to my appendix at age 67. It's possible, given our temperaments, that by the time we're totaled, we will have each other ground down to two slick steel ball bearings. Fortunately, we also navigate marriage with a bottle of steering fluid between us—half humor, half love.

I pat him above his knee, and he says, "Higher!" and leers.

The most romantic thing my husband ever said to me was just before my last birthday. "The first thing I'm going to do after your party," he said, "is make love to you, when we both are in our 70s." Wow. That's better than getting a new license plate.

More recently, lying like two spoons and enjoying the after-glow, my husband asked, "When you were young, did you ever think you'd be enjoying sex in your 70s?"

Gosh. I don't think I ever thought about it. I can remember, however, an incident when I was 40. On a home visit, I heard my parents' antique bed crash to the floor one night, an event too choice to let pass. I told my dad I was proud to have a father who could still break down his bed at 75. He blushed and laughed. My mother puffed out her cheeks and shot me a look, and then turned her head to smile.

Now I laugh, remembering that my husband turned 75 on his last birthday. But we can't hold a candle to my Great Uncle Ben and Great Aunt Maud. Story goes that Aunt

Maud went to the family doctor to ask if he couldn't give Uncle Ben saltpeter or something so he wouldn't want it every morning. The doc told Aunt Maud he wouldn't think of doing such a thing to a man who could still get it up at 92.

It's nice to know that despite high odometer readings, repairs and replacements, my family has kept its batteries charged with all gauges reading normal, normal, normal.

# Behind Closed Doors

by
Carol Commons-Brosowske

Menopause hit fast and hard. Weight gain, mood swings, hot flashes and not being able to sleep were the worst of my numerous complaints.

I had no trouble getting into a deep slumber, but like clockwork, at 2 A.M. I'd wake up and wouldn't be able to go back to sleep. Having a full-time job with little rest was really getting to me. I tried over-the-counter sleep aids, herbal tea and counting sheep. Nothing worked.

I decided to make a visit to my doctor. He prescribed Ambien. It was a new drug, a time-release capsule. It kept me asleep all night long, and I finally felt rested.

Because I was always so tired, sex had been put on the back burner. Now there were no more excuses, except we still had a teenager living at home.

The door to our bedroom stays open at all times, with an

antique quilt draped over the top of it as a decoration. The quilt is removed and put over a chair when we need privacy. The only time that quilt moved was when we wanted to get it on in the sack.

Our teenage son was on a date and wasn't expected home until later. My husband and I had a nice dinner and he cleaned up the kitchen.

There's no sexier sight than seeing a man washing dishes, so I swatted him on the butt, gave him a wink and told him, "Meet me in the boudoir in half an hour." His eyes lit up and they seemed to sparkle. I won't swear to it, but I believe I noticed some drool at the corners of his mouth.

I took a nice soak in the tub, with loads of scented bubbles, and shaved my gorilla-like legs. Since the Ambien took an hour or more to kick in, I took one while I soaked. That way, after our romp in the hay, I figured I would be ready to simply roll over and drift off into dreamland.

The next morning, I awoke before the hubby. The first thing I noticed was the door was closed and the quilt was hanging over the bedroom chair. I was confused because I didn't recall anything from the night before. *We must have had sex; there was evidence of it. Why can't I remember?* I asked myself.

Our day began like any other as we had coffee together. I didn't say a word to my husband about the night before. After all, what in the world could I say that wouldn't sound weird or as if I was ungrateful or, worse, unfulfilled? Since it was Saturday, we spent the entire day together doing yard work. Afterward, we ran some errands. I'd hoped he might jog my memory by bringing up the subject of the previous night, but he didn't. I was puzzled.

Hours later, I could no longer be silent. "Did we have sex last night?" I asked sheepishly.

"Well, yeah," he responded.

I confessed I couldn't remember and had to ask if I had been a good participant. He made it abundantly clear that I was perfect and alert every moment. "It was some of the hottest sex we've had in years. You were at your best," he remarked. "Wasn't it good for you?"

That's when I came clean. I told him about taking my sleeping pill earlier in the evening and that after that, everything was a total blur.

That night, I decided to Google the drug I had taken—there, in black and white, was the mention that the drug could cause amnesia. Aha! That's what it was. Apparently, I had missed the entire show.

I demanded an encore performance that very night. He was ready, willing and able. This time, I remembered everything . . . and if I do say so myself, we were both amazing. I waited until after the fun to take my sleeping pill.

Sleeping together took on a whole new meaning after that experience. They say one never knows what goes on behind closed doors. I don't want to ever again be the person behind that closed door who doesn't know what is going on . . . I don't want to miss out on all the fun!

# Sex and the Digital Age

Love your hard drive!

# Sending My Love

by
## Ginger Truitt

Back in the days when the Internet was new, it took a while for me to adjust. Hubby set up an email account and kept telling me how wonderful it was to be online. He would send sweet little messages and love notes to me to show just how much fun I would have.

I grew to love the Internet. I would browse for hours and send hubby little tidbits of information or interesting links. Then I discovered cyber greeting cards and spent a great deal of time picking out designs, adding my own wording and font colors and choosing musical selections. When my friends opened their cards, they were greeted with anything from a simple one-page "hello" to a multipage show of dancing bears, blooming flowers or a version of *Soul Man*.

One morning, I let the kids pick out cards to send to each of our family members and several friends. Then I decided I would send something to Hubby.

I chose a card that was six pages long and had lots of cool sound effects. The font was tiny, but grew larger until the words filled the screen and exploded into fireworks. I set out to be romantic, but then thought it would be fun to be a little naughty.

The first page shouted the promise, "Tonight's the night!"

Page 2 proclaimed that Hubby was going to have all of his fantasies fulfilled.

Pages 3, 4 and 5 gave explicit details of what he could expect throughout the evening ahead.

And Page 6 ended with the Campbell's Soup slogan, "M'm! M'm! Good!"

I reviewed the card and, pleased with my creativity, I hit *send*. I couldn't wait for his response.

When Hubby got home from work that evening, I was greeted with the usual peck on the lips. Not exactly what I expected, considering all that I had promised. Then Hubby went to check his email. I decided he must not have had a chance to go online at work and was probably just now getting my card. I waited a few minutes then casually walked into our home office.

"So, did you get anything interesting?" I asked innocently.

"Nope," he replied.

"Are you sure?" I grinned, thinking he was pulling my leg.

"No, I didn't get anything but some junk mail."

"But I sent you a card this morning!"

He shrugged casually and said, "Well, you didn't send it to me."

I began to panic. My naughty little card was somewhere out there in cyberspace! I tried to remember every person we had sent cards to that morning. All of the aunts and uncles, the pastor's wife, the kids' Sunday school teachers, and then, it hit me—my father-in-law! The children had chosen one for their grandfather, and it was the last card we sent before I designed my sexy little number for my husband.

I suddenly felt sick to my stomach. I could picture his surprised expression when he opened the card and saw all of those fireworks and exploding words that promised a night of passion. Did I mention he was a Quaker minister?

Hubby noticed the green shade creeping over my face and asked what was wrong. I told him the whole story. I gave him the details of the card and how I was sure I had mistakenly sent it to his father.

First, he gleefully asked if I was going to follow through on my promises. I gave him my death stare. Nothing ruins a romantic mood more than knowing that you just offered yourself up on a silver platter to your father-in-law!

Hubby said I should call and tell his dad not to open the card. I dialed the number and had the privilege of telling my sweet Quaker mother-in-law that I had sent her husband an erotic email. I asked her to please ask him not to open it, but it was too late. She said he had already received the card and sent a reply.

Hanging up the phone, I dashed to the computer. I was queasy with anticipation as I waited for his email to download.

I opened it and read the following: "I received your card. Have you been drinking? Thought you should know I saved it to the hard drive to show your children when they are older."

Gotta love that Quaker sense of humor. On the upside, since that fateful day, I have been able to claim the status of favorite daughter-in-law.

# Facebook Faux Pas

by
Suzette Martinez Standring

I'm wide-open to sex and shenanigans with anybody—according to my Facebook page—which came as a big surprise to me. I'm 60 years old and a syndicated religion columnist. Rather unseemly, don't you think? It all traces back to a technosaur oopsie on social media.

Here is where I went wrong. Back when I was a social-media neophyte, I set up a profile on Facebook to promote my professional writing. I wanted everything just so. Do you know how much angst that creates when having to feature "favorite musicians?" Don't get me started on choosing "favorite books." Then there was the section that asked who was I interested in: Men? Women? In my naïveté, I thought, *Now why would I limit new friends to one gender? Of course I'm interested in everybody.* So I checked both.

Little did I know I was sending the wrong signal in social

traffic; the world now saw me as cruising down the freeway of love and hogging both lanes. Yet, I had no idea. I was posting columns and "friending" new people with the aim of expanding my readership. Looking back, some guys may have interpreted my friend requests the same as if I had given them a wink-wink from a zippy red sports car and mouthed, "Buy me a drink and bring your girlfriend!"

The first inkling of my gaffe started with emails from strange men, Baby Boomers like me. They were full of flattery—"You're so pretty" and "I'd like to get to know you better."

But I dismissed them, believing a certain number of nut jobs and lonely hearts were bound to surface on Facebook. What gave me pause was the number of messages that read, "You sound *very* interesting."

*Really. That many men are interested in my religion columns?*

When I looked these guys up on Facebook, most had no personal information on their profiles. But they had women as "friends." The profile photos of such men appeared to be magazine-model handsome, supposedly rich and successful. A few so-called high-ranking officers in the military weighed in with interest. Please. I may be a technosaur, but I'm no dummy. Why would an American Army general write to me in broken English as if he had a foreign accent?

Invariably, the wink-wink-leer email would say, "Tell me your dreams. You sound like a very fun lady."

I'd get all huffy and fire back, "If you bothered to read my profile, you'd see that I am happily married."

Well, my bad. I forgot I had kept my marital status

blank to protect my husband's privacy. So there was no hint, whisper or thinly veiled reference to my beloved. It was at that moment I realized, *Who could blame the casual Facebook passers-by for thinking, "Ooh-la-la, unattached and swings both ways!"* after reading my page?

Did I tell my husband about the emails? Yes, but I won't get on my high horse about openness and trust. It's called keeping a man's "two feet in one shoe." I had shown my hubby the photo of some impossibly handsome man (no doubt faked and photo-shopped to a gorgeous extreme), and then pronounced, with great annoyance, "Can you believe this guy? He's crazy about me!" I could be wrong, but in some ways, I think my stock with my husband went up.

Upon discovering my Facebook faux pas, I unchecked "men" and "women" in the "Interested In" section, and the "wow-you-sound-*very*-interesting" emails stopped.

On some very odd level—ouch.

# For a Good Time, Call

by
Stacey Gustafson

My dalliance with phone sex came about despite the obvious warning signs and my better judgment.

I dedicated five hours each day to write and catch up on social media. Every morning, I gathered my writing journal, iPhone and coffee and shuffled upstairs to my lair. Supplies by my side, I plopped down to finish my mystery novel.

*Click, click.*

"What's this?! How come nothing's happening? I said aloud.

Usually, when I'm unable to get Internet access, I call in "The Expert," who happens to be my 16-year-old son. Since he was in school, I contacted my next-best resource.

"You free?" I asked my friend, Mary, while banging my head on the desk. "I'm on a tight deadline and my computer won't cooperate."

"I'll be right over," she said with a snort.

I dragged Mary inside before she even pressed the door-bell.

"What's going on?" she asked, yanking her arm from my grip.

"No idea. When I turn on the computer, it asks for a 16-digit password."

*Who the heck remembers passwords?!* I screamed in my head.

"Maybe your connection's loose," she said and proceed-ed to unplug and replug each cord from both the computer and printer. A few clicks later, the same message appeared on the screen: "Enter your password."

*What the hell?*

"It could be your router or modem," said Mary, looking around my desk.

*Speak English, woman. What's a router?*

"Let's find out that's what it is. Do you have a contract with your Internet provider?"

"I've called before, but they ask so many questions I usually end up frustrated," I whined. "But I'll give it a shot again."

I leafed through a pile of notes in my desk drawer and found the phone number for the technical support of our In-ternet provider, Berserk.com. For $199 per year, your ques-tions were guaranteed to be answered 24/7.

I strapped on my headset and dialed 888-IT-SUCKS. I waited on hold for an hour and was startled when I heard the connection finally pick up. "This is Jason at technical support," said a guy with a low voice and slight accent. "How are you?" Within seconds, his picture popped onto my screen.

*Live technical support? Weird.*

"Fine. You?" I answered.

*What's with the chitchat? Chop chop.*

"I'm good. Thanks for asking. How may I assist you to-day?"

"I think I have a problem with my router."

"What's going on?"

In my sloppy, low-tech way, I translated my crisis to the technician, my best friend Mary by my side for moral support. I told the tech what we had done and that my friend thought the problem must be something bigger.

"My girlfriend thinks I have a corrupt cable connection," I blurted out.

"Tell me more," he said in a slow, suggestive way.

*Why is he acting so strange?*

"She didn't notice any problems with the hook up and tried again. Nothing happened."

"No," Jason said. "Tell me more about your *girlfriend*."

"What?"

"So you have a *girlfriend*?"

*Is this guy saying what I think he's saying? I just want tech support!*

I motioned to Mary to listen in on the call. She pressed her ear against the headset and her eyes bulged.

"Yes, she's my girlfriend from the neighborhood," I said matter-of-factly.

Mary made a cuckoo motion at her temple. She whispered

to me, "Let him talk. Let's see what happens."

*Tech support, my ass.*

"How long has she been your *girlfriend*?"

"We met about five years ago."

"Is she your *lover*?" he said, smearing the last word so suggestively it sounded more like "lov-errrrrrrrrrr."

*Where are you going with this, JASON?* My mouth agape, I said nothing.

"What are you wearing?" he then said. I could almost see his leer.

I mouthed to Mary, "Pervert!"

"Will you Snap Chat me a nude picture?" he asked next.

"Hey, what's your name again?" I asked him, clenching my teeth.

"Jason."

"Where are you?"

"Delhi."

"Well, Jason, I don't think you should be talking to me this way," I said, a little too loudly. "I just need some technical support. I don't wish to deal with your sexual innuendos or have phone sex with you. Is there anyone else there I can talk to?"

The longest pause in history ricocheted through the phone lines and across the continents.

*Tick tock, buddy.*

"So sorry," he said with a stutter. "Please don't get me in trouble. Let me get back to your problem and try to fix your connection. OK?"

He gained remote access to my computer and had it up

and running in no time.

"I'm going to add six months to your contract," he said with a stammer. "Are we good now?"

"Make it a year, and I'll forget the whole thing happened," I said. He agreed. And then his icon disappeared in a puff.

Now that's what I call problem-solving!

# Perfect Match

by
Myron J. Kukla

Computer dating sites are all the rage these days among people who are too busy working to pursue the opposite sex in more traditional ways, like meeting strangers in bars and stalking.

Advertising commercials for Internet matchmaking services like eHarmony.com, match.com and russianbrides. com are everywhere. Whenever I hear an advertisement for one of these places, I am reminded of my own venture in running a computer dating service back in my college days in the early 1980s.

It all started one Friday night when I was sitting around with my friends Fred and Joe watching *Brady Bunch* reruns on TV and making rude comments about Marcia. Then a commercial came on for a computer dating service. The commercial touted the advantages of making the perfect match by way of a computer scientifically comparing your personality preferences to a database of other would-be partners.

"What pathetic kind of losers would need a computer dating service to find a date on a Friday night?" asked Fred, who had recently escorted his cousin to the winter formal and had a fondness for biting his toenails.

Joe and I looked at Fred and then at ourselves. That's when we realized we had found a market for computer dating—Friday night losers.

Within a half-hour, we had sketched out plans to start a computer dating service at our college. Fred would handle the computer matching because he had a Radio Shack TRS-80 and a spreadsheet. Joe—a psychology major—would put the profile questionnaire together. My job was to handle the advertising in the student newspaper.

Three weeks later, we ran our first series of ads. "Tired of sitting around the dorm by yourself on Friday nights? Now, Scientific Computer Dating Service can get you the dates you've been missing. You'll get the names and phone numbers of people who match your profile, every week."

By the next Monday, 24 students had forked out $30 for us to help them find their dream partner. They sent the money to a post office box, and we sent them personality profiles to fill out. The questionnaires were just a formality, however. In our first batch of applicants, we had 21 guys signing up and three girls. It didn't take a computer to figure out that each girl was going to get calls from 21 guys for dates.

So, we ran another batch of ads to even out the numbers, but no girls signed up. Instead, another two dozen guys did!

Now, each of the three girls using our computer dating services would be getting calls for dates from 45 different guys.

In the meantime, the first batch of guys started writing letters to us complaining that we kept sending the names of the same three girls each week. Frantic about what to do, we misspelled and altered those girls' names so they looked like different co-eds on paper.

We lucked out on the third set of ads—another girl signed on. But another two dozen more guys joined, as well. The original three girls, and the newbie, were now being barraged hourly by 80 companionship-crazed guys calling them for dates.

Eventually, the three girls began writing letters of complaint about our service and demanding their money back. We wouldn't reply. We just kept sending their names to the same guys on our lists and others who had signed up.

That's when the three girls revolted. One of them offered to pay us to drop her name from this list, another said she was getting married, and the third wrote us she had died and would no longer need our services. But we ignored their pathetic pleading letters and kept sending the ladies' names to an increasing number of college guys who kept signing up for the promised perfect match.

This was strange because we had stopped advertising. Even without advertising, we kept getting more and more applications coming in from guys every week, and none of them were complaining any more. It was then we realized that we hadn't gotten a single complaint from the fourth girl who had signed up for computer dating.

Curious, we called up "Heidi," our uncomplaining client, and found out why she had no complaints. Heidi was a hooker who had evidently been keeping our male clients happy.

The information produced a moral dilemma for us. Unknowingly, we were involved in a prostitution ring, something that was obviously against campus rules and the law and could get us arrested. On the other hand, Heidi offered to cut us in on part of her take if we kept the computer dating service going.

In the end, Joe and I got out of that business, completed our college degrees and went on to become upstanding citizens. The last we heard of Fred and Heidi, they had moved to California where they were running a successful computer dating service.

# Cyber Cherry

by
## Charlotta Ladoo

I leaned back in my chair and wiped my mouth with a paper napkin. "I'm stuffed. I really shouldn't have eaten that last piece of pizza."

Francine let out a sigh. "Oh please, you eat like a bird. Angelino's Pizza is the best. Now come on, don't keep me in the dark any longer. When we were at work today, you said you had something important to show me tonight."

I shot to my feet and took the dishes to the sink, rinsed them and put them in the dishwasher. I was stalling, wishing I had never said anything to Francine. Now I felt really embarrassed about what I'd done, and a little ashamed. *Normal people don't have to resort to this*, I thought to myself.

With nothing else left to do, I gave in. "OK, I guess now is as good a time as any to reveal my big secret. Come."

I led her down the hall to my den. I booted up the computer and navigated to an Internet dating site. As soon as the sign-on screen popped up, Francine said, "You didn't . . . really . . . did you?" She plopped down in a chair and leaned closer to the monitor for a better look. The screen was filled with thumbnails of men, photos so small she had to squint. "You put a profile on here?"

Still embarrassed, I became defensive. "I'm tired of waiting for the right one to come along. I'm 29 years old and still haven't . . . " I stopped myself. "How else am I going to meet someone? There isn't one single guy at our church—they're all married. It's not like I'm going to find Mr. Right in a bar. We've seen how well that works. Remember last weekend when we went out with Cindi and Dee? Well, let's just say I'm getting very tired of watching other women get all the attention. This seemed like a logical alternative." I was nothing if not logical. Dr. Spock was my role model—not the baby doctor Spock, but the Vulcan.

"Have you thought this through? I hear there are a lot of weirdoes on these websites," Francine said, running her fingers through her dark hair.

"I just started, but it seems harmless enough. Check out these profiles—pages and pages of them. There are some normal-looking men on here." My chewed fingernails danced across the keyboard as I flipped through the screens with practiced ease. "See, you can narrow your search by location or age or any other factor you're looking for. There's even an instant-chat feature."

Just as the words left my mouth, the computer made a soft *ding*, and a chat box popped up. *From loverboy: Hey beautiful, what you doin'?*

Francine jumped as if she'd been hit by 2,000 volts. "Holy cow! Now what do we do?"

"We can chat or decline. But let's have some fun. I'll show you his profile."

"He's cute," Francine said, quickly reading his bio. "He lives about an hour away. And he's the right age."

Another *ding*.

*From loverboy: Hey doll, you there?*

I began to answer then hesitated. "I don't know about this. I was on here the other night, and some guys just wanted to talk dirty." A nervous giggle escaped. "I was hoping to find someone I actually wanted to meet, but that hasn't happened yet. So last night I figured, what the heck."

Francine was so flabbergasted she almost fell off her chair. "You had cybersex?"

"Is that what they call it? Don't look at me like that. It really is harmless."

*From loverboy: you there spacecadet?*

I steeled myself and typed, Y*es, what's up with you tonight?*

Francine laughed and pointed at the screen, "You're name is 'spacecadet 6969.' I can't believe this!"

I laughed, too. "I don't know what came over me. It seemed like the thing to do. It's fun being naughty for the first time in my life."

*From loverboy: Oh darling I can't believe you asked me that . . . you know I'm up and hard for you. After last night I've been looking for you to cum back online.*

Francine looked at me, and I could tell she was wondering who this woman was and what she'd done to her friend. "Last night? You chatted with him last night? Are you going to meet him?"

I typed. *I'm here. So you liked last night?*

I said to Francine, "Oh, heavens no. I could never face him after the session we had."

She sputtered. "Wh . . . what did you *do* last night?"

"I didn't *do* anything. I just typed."

*From loverboy: You bet. I quit smoking three years ago, but it felt like I needed a cigarette after our chat. So when can we meet so I can do all the things we talked about last night in person?*

"Uh oh, looks like trouble," said Francine.

"Oh, come on now. It's not as if he can reach through the computer and get me or anything. What should we say?" I chewed a fingernail.

"We?"

"Unwind a little. Type something to him. I'll go get us some wine."

"Wine? You drink at home now?"

"Cindi, from work, told me about this fantastic vintage. You'll love it."

Francine typed. *So busy this week, maybe next?*

I returned with the wine and looked at the screen. "Are you crazy? I'm never going to actually meet this guy. That would be dangerous."

"I get that, but I thought we had to string him along."

I sipped my wine and contemplated as the screen chimed again. *From loverboy: I guess I'll have to wait. I know it will be worth it.*

Francine took a deep breath and typed. *I can hardly wait to meet you.* She paused, trying to think of something seductive.

*I savor the idea of your first kiss.* She hit *send.*

I giggled. The wine was kicking in already. "Savoring the idea? You sound like a romance novel. Guys don't work that way. You've got to be more graphic, or they won't get it." I pulled the keyboard onto my lap and typed. *My tongue shyly explores your mouth.* I hit *send* and cackled like a large egg was on its way.

We waited. "Was this guy this slow last night?" Francine asked.

"Yeah, he types slow. Probably a one-handed typist."

"What do you mean, 'one handed'?"

I made a jack-off motion with my hand in my lap.

Francine put her hands to her face Macaulay-Culkin style and said, "No."

We both burst out laughing.

The computer dinged. *From loverboy: I pull you into my arms and you surrender.*

"I notice he jumps to the 'surrender' part pretty fast," Francine said as she typed. *I feel your rock hard pectoral muscles against my firm breasts.*

I smirked. "Now you're getting it, but *pectoral muscles* seems too clinical."

*From loverboy: I grab your ass and thrust my toungue deep into your mouth.*

Francine pointed at the computer and laughed again. "What a moron. He can't even spell 'tongue.'"

"You see, that's another reason I have *no* interest in meeting him."

"Oh, besides the fact that he gets his jollies online?"

"That, too."

I interlaced my fingers and thrust out my arms to crack my knuckles. "OK, this poor schmuck won't know what hit him." I typed. *I respond eagerly, hungry for your body.*

Francine said, "That was pretty lame. I thought you were going to get him going." She grabbed the keyboard and typed. *You grind your hard penis against my pubis.* She took a big gulp of her wine as she hit *send.*

We were laughing so hard, I yelled, "Stop, I've gotta pee!" When I came back into the room, loverboy still hadn't responded.

We sipped our wine, wringing the last drops out of the bottle. Eventually, the computer dinged again

*From loverboy: OMG you are so hot tonight. I want you now for real.*

We exploded into peals of laughter. When we'd recovered, we both reached for the keyboard at the same time, but I won. The house always wins. *OMG I'm so hot for you. I want to feel your body against mine.*

More laughter filled the room.

"I think we need a refill on the wine." I went to the kitchen. Just as I came back, *ding* went the computer.

*From loverboy: I want you. I want to suck your nippls and make you scream.*

"Real rocket scientist, this one," I said. "He can't even spell 'nipples.'"

Francine typed. *I nibble your earlobes.*

I pulled the keyboard away. "Come on. If we're going to play with this guy, let's really get him going." I typed. *I grab your shirt and rip it open, buttons flying.*

"Oh no, you didn't."

"Oh yes, I did." I hit *send* with a flourish.

We waited even longer this time. I fidgeted with the buttons on my sweater. "He must be typing a novel."

*From loverboy: I do the same.*

Francine said, "My, my. This guy really is a mental deficient, all this time to type that?"

I typed. *You plant kisses along the delicate lace edge of my bra.* I turned to Francine with a lopsided smile. "That ought to stimulate him."

This time, he typed a little faster. *I unhook your bra and cup your large tittys sucking on the mipples.*

We roared. "The mipples? This guy is too much."

Francine took her turn. "This is fun. I see why people do this." Typing. *I gasp. Grabbing your buttocks and pulling you against me.* She hit *send*.

I laughed. "Too lame." Grabbing the keyboard, I typed. *I can feel your erection through the material of your pants.*

We sipped our wine as we waited for his reply.

*From loverboy: I unbuckle my pants and let them fall. You drop to your knees and suck me.*

"Oh my, he's getting right to the meat of the matter," I said.

We were laughing so hard that Francine could barely get words out. "*Meat of the matter?* You crack me up. Now what?

Francine pulled off her glasses and wiped the tears from her eyes. Putting her glasses back on, she typed. *I gag.* We both roared with laughter again.

I grabbed the keyboard before Francine could hit send and backspaced over her comment. "No, no guys don't want to hear that. We've got to type something sexy, something erotic."

I pondered my response. Then it came to me.

*You're so big, it hardly fits in my mouth.* I hit the *send* button. "That's what they want to hear. He's probably sitting in his parents' basement, holding onto his four-inch pencil dick, but this is what he wants to believe could happen. The Internet is all about illusion. In *World of Warcraft*, I'm a blood elf, and here, I'm a slut. It's really no different. I have no intentions of ever meeting this guy."

Francine laughed. "You, a slut? That's as likely as your transit to the moon." She sipped her wine. "This wine is good. I think I'm getting drunk. You said you chatted with this guy last night. How'd it go?"

"We teased a little, but nothing this graphic," I said as I twirled my hair.

*From loverboy: I hold your head and f_ _k your face.*

We gasped. "We're too graphic now."

"Ewww," Francine said, grossed out. "Oh yeah, male fantasy all right. Can't even get any decent foreplay online."

"Well, what can you say after that?" I said, hitting the button to end the chat. With great gusto, I raised my wineglass and made a toast. "Here's to popping our cyber-cherries."

"Oh, that was just cunnilingus; it doesn't count," Francine said. "Remember, Bill Clinton set the new standards."

# CHAPTER SEVEN

# Afraid to Ask . . .

---

. . . but I will, anyway.

---

# Do You Vajazzle?

by
Kelly Melang

Sometimes you are taught things that stick with you, or, should I say, stick *on* you. Recently, I learned about "vajazzling" and I thought you, dear reader, could help me process this information.

Vajazzling is a new form of body art where decorative jewels are fastened to the female genitalia and vagina. So here's where I'm a little stuck—pun intended.

I pondered how one sticks the beads to the vagina—more accurately, the labia, but I guess "labiazzle" doesn't have the same ring. Are they Super Glued into place and, therefore, they have a shorter shelf life, staying in place only temporarily? Or are they permanently attached so that one day, due to age or gravity, that beautiful butterfly vajazzle turns into a hawk with a fish hanging from its beak?

*Are the beads smooth?* I wondered. *If they are real gems, with edges, will they get stuck on stuff? What if you have to go to the bathroom badly and your panties become stuck in your vajazzle—what then? Do you rip them off or just "vijizzle" in your vajazzle? And what about the fun we ladies like to have—you know, foreplay? Would you—or your partner—be cut by the jewels? And if a jewel were to fall off during the fun—and if that jewel had value—who'd get to keep it?*

I assume from the pictures I've seen that vajazzling requires the woman to have no hair . . . down there. If you got smooth as a baby's bottom for your vajazzling session, I wondered how you would stay smooth. Tweezers instead of a razor? For those of us who prefer to keep the hair, I thought it would be cool to create a vajazzle with little jeweled fairies peeking out of the bushes. I could become rich from that idea!

And yet, I wondered about the single girl and the vajazzle. How would she explain this to the new man in her life? Would she announce with great gusto, "Prepare to be dazzled!" The same could be said for newlyweds. Pondering this situation, I imagined the groom's reaction on the couple's wedding night when his bride shows him her vajazzle of "Just Married!"

I had more questions. How long would it take to be vajazzled? I so enjoy my time at the OB-GYN, with my feet aimed at the ceiling and everything showing, that I wondered if I really needed to spend hours with a stranger staring intently at my hoohee and  attaching little jewels.

Here's another question I pondered: Could I vajazzle myself? I'd have to be upside down to get it right. I'd vajazzle the word "SWIMS" because it would look the same from either direction! But how would I appropriately use that word in a vagina decoration?

And I wondered how someone came up with vajazzling to begin with. Did someone, while naked, look at her bedazzle kit and then at her vagina and think, " I need to staple a few of these beads there. Wouldn't THAT be FUN?"

Whenever an exciting new trend surfaces, I'm reminded that I am getting old. I think my vagina looks pretty good as is. I don't need to vagina-ercize it into shape, nor do I need to vajazzle a few wrinkles. I am lucky to have a great man in my life who thinks my personality sparkles enough.

But I can't help but think—what's next?

Boobazzling? Tittazzling? I can hardly wait to see.

# Booby Prize

by
## Sherri Kuhn

Breasts. Boobs, hooters, honkers, gazongas, mounds, melons, fun bags, happy sacks, rack, chest.

Whatever you call them, they're just another body part.

They fill out our sweaters, feed our babies, catch crumbs from our lunch. They attempt to defy gravity, attract attention, swell when we're hormonal and distinguish us from men—usually. And whether we're quite small up top or rather well endowed, we all have very deep feelings about our girls.

Unfortunately, my lunch crumbs fall directly onto my lap. I know all about the Wonderbra and the Itty Bitty Titty Committee, and I know that Victoria's real "secret" is just extra padding. I also know that clever way to hug myself with my arms crossed, giving me instant cleavage.

I usually don't spend a lot of time worrying about mine.

We coexist just fine—most of the time. Not counting swimsuit season.

So while I have boobs, I didn't think about them too much . . . until my seventh-grade daughter came home from school one day freaking out about boobs. Her science class was starting the reproductive health unit, and to kick it off, the girls had to watch a video on breast self-exams.

It sounded informative. It was useful information we should all know. And it was way better than the video the class was going to see the following week of a woman giving birth, which I think is perfect birth control, by the way.

"So what's the problem with the breast self-exam video?" I asked her.

"The woman in the video was *old*. Maybe even older than *you*," she answered. "With huge, saggy boobs that looked like pancakes."

Obviously, my daughter had no idea things could get to that point. No clue. Apparently, I hadn't had the proper breast discussion with her, beyond simply telling her that yes, she would get boobs and no, they wouldn't be big. For her, it was like finding out the Tooth Fairy, the Easter Bunny and Santa Claus were all frauds; that candy really is bad for your teeth, or that you really can't be an astronaut without understanding algebra. A small bit of hope for the future was lost right there in science class, Room 14, second period. She was terrified of the prospect of one day having boobs that would look like plastic grocery bags full of JELL-O pudding—just hanging there.

"Couldn't they have hired someone with *normal* boobs,

Mom? Someone younger? Ugh, it was disgusting!"

So we had a long conversation about normal and how the models strewn throughout *InStyle* magazine weren't representative of the population in general.

And how she's got genetics on her side.

When your mother is a card-carrying member of the Itty Bitty Titty Committee, there are some things you'll just never need to worry about.

As long as you have a Victoria's Secret charge card, that is.

# Wet Dreams

by
Connie E. Curry

The wonders of a mother and her versatility are amazing. As a mother, I can conduct an intelligent conversation, answer the door and take the cookies out of the oven before the smoke detector goes off, all at the same time. I can do dishes, listen to a child read and even stir the muffin mix as I answer a ringing telephone. I know when the family is down to three Q-tips, how many slices of bread are left and who needs new razor blades and for which razor. Most importantly, I know when to buy these items before they are totally gone.

I can also find lost items, even when I didn't misplace them. For example, those that I adore and live with can never find the ketchup. My husband can spot a deer 15 miles away between cornrows with the naked eye while driving 50 mph, but he can't see the ketchup bottle on the front shelf in the refrigerator.

And I am a qualified homework assistant—a pro, as a matter of fact. I have refreshed my memory on fractions, proper grammar, how gravity works and where Israel is located on a map. But just when I think I am the top dog in this home, my ego gets squashed.

My son, Ryan, brought home a school assignment. Like so many other times, I was ready to gather my scruples and assist him.

He removed his homework from his backpack and sat down at the kitchen table. While peeling potatoes, I peered over him at his homework. I so hoped it wasn't a science assignment—science always put me into a whirlwind of mass confusion and made me feel stupid. I was a Super Mom who could do almost anything. I could catch baseballs, drive a standard transmission automobile and hammer nails into a wall to hang a picture. When it came to science, I knew it was Isaac Newton who discovered gravity. Wasn't it something to do with an apple falling from a tree? However, just for the record, I learned all these things and more in a previous time, 20 years ago. My memory bank was growing poor.

I looked again at his assignment. He was to define 20 words. "Piece of cake, Ryan. This isn't a difficult assignment," I said.

"But Mom, I don't understand these words. I can't even pronounce them!"

"Ryan, please don't complain. I know you just want to go outside to play, but you must do your homework first."

As I looked more closely at his vocabulary words, my

jaw dropped. "Orgasm, masturbation, ovulation, hormones, uterus, conception, sexual intercourse . . ." Then I saw it! "Wet dream."

*WET DREAM! And they call this health class!* I screamed in my head.

I felt myself panic. *Why do I have to get dinner and help with this homework assignment?* I thought. *Isn't this a guy thing? Where's my husband when I need him?*

And I couldn't understand why "wet dream" was one of the words to be defined. *Isn't that slang? I'll bet the farm that wet dream isn't in my Webster's Dictionary.*

My motherly internal ramblings continued. *Why does my sweet, innocent child need to learn these words now? He likes crayons, cartoons and Pop Tarts. And he thinks girls are stupid.*

With all that said—to myself, of course—and after much consideration, thought and confidence in the teaching staff, I concluded that they knew what was best for my child. It was time to teach Ryan some facts about life. So, as discreetly as I could without being too technical, I helped him define each word and tried to simplify my answers when he asked questions.

When we arrived at the words "wet dream," I skimmed through the worksheet.

He said, "Oh, heck, Mom. I know this one! I do that all the time!"

I looked out the window to see if his father was coming home. I sighed, my heart raced and I kept in mind what celebrity sex therapist Dr. Ruth Westheimer always said: "Masturbation is normal and healthy." Therefore, in a calm voice,

I simply replied, "Oh, you do? Well, I guess you don't need my help on finding the definition."

I turned to finish dinner and tried not to cry. I wanted to peel a very juicy onion to give me an excuse for the tears forming in my eyes. I wanted Ryan to be in diapers and crawling again. I wanted his father home—now!

Done with his homework, Ryan darted outside to play. I quickly looked at the definition he had written. It read, "Wet dream: When you slobber on your pillowcase during the night while sleeping."

I breathed a sigh of relief.

Who said Dr. Ruth knows everything?

# Drugstore Jive

by
### Darlene Cobb

When I was 18 years old, I worked as a part-time sales clerk at a local drugstore. I was saving money to go to college and was very innocent about anything related to sex.

A great example is the customer who wanted to buy condoms. I had to ask another clerk what he really wanted, since I thought condoms had something to do with condo homes. The clerk smiled then whispered to me as she pointed to the shelf, "He wants rubbers, but not the kind for your feet!"

Another time, a guy asked for prophylactics. I thought that had something to do with athletic equipment. Of course, I guessed wrong.

Some men would come into the store and ask for Trojans. *Hmm, do they want a book about the Trojan War or maybe some sports-team item?* I'd ask myself while trying to figure out how to best help them. *There are quite a few teams called "The Trojans."*

I soon found out not only were there Trojan condoms,

but Trojan vibrators, as well. Oh, that was another area that confused me: whenever a customer asked for anything that vibrated, all I could think of was something to relax muscles. I guess in a way, I was correct.

One day, a lady asked for rubbers. With her being a woman, I figured she would want something in rain-protection wear, not condoms. Boy, was I wrong! She did, in fact, want condoms. I couldn't believe that a female would ask for something that males usually purchased.

I had another man with a full head of hair ask for Preparation H, so I took him to the hair section. He grinned and said to me, "Wrong end!" There again, I had to get help from another clerk since I obviously didn't know which end was up!

When a female customer wanted to buy K-Y Jelly, I just knew it had to be in the food department. Well, I soon found out you don't eat this kind of jelly! And then there was the lady who came into the drugstore looking for Ben Wa balls. I escorted her to the children's toy section.

When we got there, she started laughing and loudly asked, "Don't you have a sex-toy department?"

My face turned red as I replied, "I don't think so, but I'll ask." At least I was right. We didn't have a sex-toy department, but the store did carry a few related items. And no, we didn't have the balls she wanted.

I'll never forget the time a lady with bright orange hair and wearing a yellow dress came into the store and wandered up and down the aisles. I approached her and asked, "Can I help you?"

She said, "I need a teat dilator."

Wanting to appear knowledgeable, I brought out a breast pump.

The lady exclaimed loudly, "No, honey. It's for cow teats!"

I received a valuable education working at the drugstore. But as we all know, the meaning of words often changes. Take, for instance, the word "thong." It used to mean flip-flop shoes. Now I'm told a thong is underwear or a swimsuit bottom.

I'm glad I don't have to work in a drugstore anymore.

# Nothing Else to be Said

by
Candy Schock

Eleven-year-old Melissa ran into the kitchen where I was preparing dinner. Home from school, she dropped her book bag on the floor, slid out of her shoes and sat down at the kitchen table.

"Hi, honey. How was your day?" I asked. I opened the refrigerator, took out an apple for her and poured her a glass of milk.

"Ah, Mom. Chris's mom lets her have a bread and jelly sandwich and pop," she said, whining.

It was the same argument every day after school. I had finally learned not to respond with the typical, "If she let Chris jump off a bridge . . . ?" So I ignored her taunt.

Realizing she was not about to get her way, my daughter changed the subject. "Mrs. Armstrong said I was tops in my reading group."

"That's wonderful, Melissa. Daddy and I are very proud

of you." I rinsed some cauliflower in the sink and grabbed a large knife to cut it up.

"Bradley said a bad word today in school," she then said, offhandedly. She was now sporting a milk mustache.

"Oh?"

"Yeah, he said . . . ah, can I say it without getting in trouble?"

"What does the word start with?" I asked, not wanting to set a precedent. I opened the silverware drawer and counted out four knives, forks and spoons.

"It was the F-word!" she exclaimed, in such a tone that it was as if the world was coming to an end. "Mrs. Armstrong sent him to the principal's office. Boy, his mom is going to KILL him!"

*Maybe it is the end of the world—at least for Bradley*, I thought. I tried not to become annoyed. After all, Melissa had certainly heard the word before on the playground and other places beyond my control. But I hated to think it was part of a fourth-grader's reality. Was I being naïve?

Placing the silverware onto the table, Melissa jumped up, turning over the chair. She righted it then began setting the table without my asking.

I opened the oven and stirred the casserole, smiling to myself. *She is growing up.*

Now cutting potatoes, I was surprised when Melissa asked, "Hey, Mom, what's does 'an erection' mean?"

The knife slipped off the potato I was quartering and I cut myself. A drop of blood fell into the sink and stained the peelings a pretty red.

Melissa and I had had "the talk" several months ago. As a registered nurse, I had prided myself on knowing the anatomy and all the correct words. But wanting to be sure I handled this significant parental responsibility well, I had searched online for the best ways to explain grown-up concepts to an 11-year- old. After all, it wasn't just a matter of anatomy and "how-to." I wanted to convey to Melissa the specialness and closeness of sex. And I wanted her to grow up thinking about sex as something to be experienced at the right time.

I quickly dropped the knife into the sink, wiped my bloody finger on a towel and pulled out a chair for her to sit on, which she did. Melissa looked up at me expectantly.

"Well, Melissa, remember I explained to you that when a man is with someone special who he loves, sometimes blood flows into his penis and makes it very hard so that . . ."

Melissa jumped out of the chair, knocking it over again, and waved a dismissive hand at me. "Oh, Mom!" she said, laughing with contempt. "You mean a 'boner.'"

And with that, Melissa ran from the kitchen, nimbly avoiding the fallen chair and leaping over her shoes and book bag. I could only stand there nonplussed, not wanting to accept the obvious. My little girl was indeed growing up. I stifled a long sigh.

Then I picked up the paring knife again. For there was nothing else to be said.

# Creating a
# Sex Goddess

by
Siobhan McKinney

Men never seem to appreciate the work that goes into creating a sex goddess—all they ever see is the finished product. I guess we women make it look easy, but it's not.

I live in the United Kingdom and admit I have high standards. But cutbacks at work meant I needed to cut back on little luxuries, too. Not that I look upon my salon time as a luxury. It really is a necessity. I like to look good for my partner as much as for myself. If stubbly legs and ingrown hairs along the bikini line make me dry heave, what must my man think? Besides, I like soft, smooth skin. It feels so much . . . cleaner.

It is not easy being a sex goddess. Waxing, manicures, hairdressers, spray tan, pedicure—hell, it all mounts up. And the products and prices required to maintain this look border on ridiculous. I should have seen the future and bought shares in one of the big name brands or trained as a beauty therapist. I don't think I'm therapist material, though. Making a living ripping the hair off a stranger's hoo-ha is not my idea of a solid career move. Besides, my attempt at home treatment was a consummate failure.

I will never try to wax my bikini area myself again.

Never.

Disaster.

Explanation: Per the instructions, I heated the wax in the microwave. Of course, it was too damned hot to apply. Testing it with my finger occasionally to see if the magma's intensity had lowered, I yelped, hollered and jumped around as I waited for the wax to cool. Three blisters later, it seemed suitable for application.

God really made it awkward to self-apply wax to your nether regions. You either straddle a mirror or somehow organize your legs so you can see what's going on. Anyway, sometime later—job done. The area was coated in a thick layer of "fresh peach melon" wax.

But, from the pain of the first dollop, I began to wonder if its removal would tear off a hunk of flesh. I chickened out. I know, I know—dumb move. But this was my first, and only, time. So there I was, with only half of my lady parts covered in wax.

I ran a bath, in hopes the wax would soften after soaking in it, and that I would then be able to rub it off. Rookie mistake. It didn't work. Then I thought, *Hey, it'll wear off.* So, I toweled myself and yeah, all the towel fluff stuck to me.

What to do now? Deciding I needed to go ahead and yank the wax off, I sat down on the loo seat to muster up some courage for the main event. I got stuck to the seat. Stuck to the seat! No phone nearby. Who would I call anyway? I was naked and stuck to a loo seat.

I was only half-covered in wax and realized that if I was going to rip it off, I should do it all to do the job right. Can't have a half wax, can I? So I applied the rest of the warm wax as I sat on the loo seat. Not a good idea. Some trickled further back and it set around my bum hole and lady lips. I'd sealed myself shut. Could this get any worse?

Eventually, I bit the bullet. I turned myself into a contortionist, using one hand to steady myself against the wall and the other to remove the wax. I managed to rip a hair carpet and half my bits off.

The sacrifices we ladies make. A woman's work is never done. I spend hours in the gym flashing my whitened smile, followed by a pore-cleansing sauna, and then exfoliation, depilation and moisturizing to prevent dehydration all over. I must maintain my pumiced heels and painted toenails, tidy cuticles and manicured talons. Men have no idea the time it takes to artfully fix my glossy mane with tumbling curls to frame my face, just so, or to add another tousle or two.

From top to toe the work continues, blemishes are disguised and assets are accentuated with cosmetic expertise gleaned from magazines. I've learned to apply a brush of shadow on my cleavage above the chicken filets in my pushup bra. I buy fat pants in the sexiest designs that hide cellulite, muffin tops and wobbly thighs. All so I can have eye-catching curves and a smooth silhouette. I wear high-heeled shoes that cripple my feet, but make my booty look good in this dress, that skirt, those slacks. Oh, God! I've got nothing to wear.

Meanwhile, men shower, shave, have a shit. They dress in chinos, belted below their paunch, and a polo shirt that highlights their jowls. Before going out the door, they check—spectacles, testicles, car keys and wallet. They fart, smile and scratch their balls. They're good to go.

Next time, I want to be a man.

# Just Add Water

---

Keeping it wet.

---

# Rockin' the Love Boat

by
Kathleene Baker

I'd been divorced about a year and had absolutely no interest in men. Naturally, that's when one nudged his way into my life. However, I took it slow—very slow, much to Jerry's chagrin. At evening's end, we'd share a few long, romantic kisses at my front door, and I'd nonchalantly send him on his way. Not used to such treatment, the handsome Marine from Texas was bamboozled. Even though I chose to close the door, it was self-imposed agony for me. Yet I knew it was even more frustrating for him, and it was so worth it!

Several months later, in the midst of a God-awful Kansas heat wave, we headed to Texas for a long weekend of swimming, fishing and visiting with Jerry's parents at their lake house. I'd met them once prior and found time spent with his mom, Iva, was like hanging out with a girlfriend. I adored them both. They were more fun than most of our friends.

At the time, I was 29, and Jerry was 35. Being such avant-garde parents, I'm sure they expected we would sleep together. Wrong! Out of respect for them, I chose to have my own room—with no middle-of-the-night visits allowed. I even locked the door. Again, that good-looking Marine was rendered speechless. I came to love the game of cat and mouse, because it made for mind-blowing sexual encounters when he least expected.

While at the lake house, Jerry and I transformed the bass boat into a sex-mobile. On stifling afternoons, I'd purr and bat my eyelashes at him. "I'm about ready to go for a ride and a swim."

"Sounds good to me, too. It's hot as hell!" The Marine usually gave me a wink, and I swear he'd begin to pant before we were out of the house.

Texas nights are gorgeous, and black skies hang heavy with silver stars. Temperatures remain warm, making nudity more than comfortable. And the sway of the boat enhanced our activities.

Late one night, just as things were heating up in that boat, I arched my back, raised my derriere and mumbled, "Oh, my God!"

I tried to calm myself and relax, but then I began arching and thrashing about again. "Oh, my God! OH, MY GOD!"

Amazed, Jerry whispered, "Good grief—already? Wow!"

"NO. Not already. Not WOW. And maybe not ever again!" I pushed him off me.

"What? Did I hurt you? What's wrong? You're quivering."

"I've been snake bit, on my left cheek and more than once. Damn, what a way to die—and right before the magic moment."

Jerry grabbed the flashlight, filled with nearly dead batteries, and found no sign of a snake in the boat. But he did make out marks on my fanny!

I screeched, "If it was a baby snake, we'll never find it. We've got to get back to the house. You know a baby's venom is more dangerous than that of a grown snake and this lake crawls with copperheads and cottonmouths. What the hell were we thinking coming out here at night?"

The motor on that boat sounded as if it might fly apart as we sped across the lake. My heart raced as I fumbled, trying to dress myself. I gasped for breath and didn't know if it was from fright or the venom taking effect. Being miles from a town—let alone a doctor—I was terrified.

Jerry's parents heard us barrel into the house and came charging from their bedroom, still hurriedly wrapping robes about themselves, to see what the commotion was all about.

His mom whimpered, "Oh, dear Lord," and grabbed me as I began to cry.

Between sobs, I choked out, "I've been snake bit . . . I know I'm going to die!"

Oran, Jerry's burly Marine Corps Dad, was the only one who remained calm and levelheaded. "OK, before we take off for the hospital, we need to know what we're dealing with. I've seen plenty of snake bites—and it could have been something else. Possibly a spider. Little darlin', I need to see those bites." His deep southern drawl was demanding.

"What? You're going to look at my butt? Are you shitting me?!" I said, stunned.

Jerry laid a calming hand on my shoulder. "Kathy, we have no choice. Go lie on the bed and pull down your britches. Just do it! This is no time to act the prima donna." I discovered Jerry could be just as bossy as his dad.

"Holy crap, someone just shoot me now!" I shouted and stomped to the bedroom.

Iva followed me with some towels and draped my rearend like I was about to have surgery. God bless that woman.

Oran donned his reading glasses and bent over to study my wounds. Mercy, he even touched me a few times. I tried to tell myself, *Hey, it's just another good-looking Marine pawing around on my behind.* Then I snapped, "WHY are you touching me?!"

"Feeling for swelling and fever and checking the edges of these punctures. Some are uniform while others appear a little jagged. I'm just trying to help. Trust me."

It seemed like an eternity before he announced I'd not been bitten by a snake, of that he was positive. But not knowing what my problem was, he grabbed a light capable of beaming into the next county. "Come on, Jerry! We're going to inspect the boat."

Meanwhile, Iva cleaned and disinfected my cheek with her favorite cure-all, Dr. Tichenor's Antiseptic. I'd never heard of the stuff and swear it must have originally been sold from medicine wagons. The bottle and label appeared exactly like the ones seen in old Westerns. When she finished, I considered guzzling the contents to calm my frenzied nerves.

I sat apprehensively on the couch as Iva handed me another glass of wine. I'd thrown down the first glass in two gulps.

Then I heard the guys laughing as they came up to the house, which ticked me off immediately. *Even if a spider had nibbled on my ass, it could easily have been poisonous.*

The guys walked into the living room and stood in front of me with smirks on their faces. Oran spoke. "We found the culprit. Catch!"

I faintly felt something hit my lap as I shot straight into the air. I knew it was going to be a dead baby snake. Their behavior told me all I needed to know. I wasn't in danger, but their antics still sucked.

When my feet were back on the floor, no baby snake was anywhere to be seen. I frantically brushed my hands down the front of my clothing. *Were they stupid enough to bring that sucker back alive?* I wondered. *Is it on the loose again?*

"I don't see a thing, boys." I glared at them both.

Oran handed me his flashlight and told me to glance about the floor. Ha! A couple of small fishhooks glinted in the light. *Fishhooks? Fricking fishhooks?!*

"Do you remember dropping some hooks this morning when we were gearing up to fish for crappie?" Oran asked.

Obviously, I'd missed retrieving a few, and they'd slipped into the vinyl folds of the boat seat. They were new, with no rust; I would live to rock the boat another day.

Oran looked at me seriously. "And now, Iva and I are going back to bed to pick up where we left off—you know, before you two blasted into the house like a SWAT team."

"Jerry, take that whacked-out Kansas woman to bed, for God's sake!" Oran said. "If you're smart, you'll take care of her in the best way you know how. As in—the finest performance of your lifetime! Oh, and if you thought we bought your fishing story earlier, we aren't stupid. It was pitiful."

Answering for my stunned boyfriend, I spun on my heel, stood up straight and saluted the man who would one day become my father-in-law. "Yes, sir! Anything else, sir?"

"Carry on, darlin' . . . and enjoy." Then he winked at me—just like his son!

# Slippery When Wet

by
Shari Courter

When our kids were young and my husband, Ron, worked nights, we had to be creative when it came to our sex life. Whenever they asked us about the squeaky noises coming from upstairs in the middle of the day, we blamed it on a squirrel in the attic. Our lovemaking usually happened while they watched episodes of *Barney the Dinosaur,* and let's be honest, most of the time the squeaking never actually lasted one full episode.

Their questions about the squirrel and the squeaking during the daytime became more frequent. That's when Ron and I made our stupidest adult decision ever, a decision so bad it will go down in history. We bought a waterbed.

Suddenly, the kids were asking why they heard our bed "splashing." We blamed it on our "wrestling." Yes, our kids grew up thinking we wrestled. Don't judge—it's all we could come up with during a moment of panic, out of breath between sloshes, as they stood knocking on our door one day. "And no, you can't watch," usually followed the, "We're just wrestling" comment.

Clearly, we didn't think the whole waterbed thing through. And while we're on the topic of not thinking things through, let's discuss the evening Ron and I actually broke the waterbed, um, wrestling.

That baffling realization occurred in the heat of the moment when we were both getting wet—more wet than normal. Our confused eyes met. As we were left riding the remainder of the wave until the mattress came to a complete stop, our minds simultaneously connected the dots of what had just happened.

Oh, crap.

We jumped out of bed in a flurry of accusations. The line between passion and throwing each other under the bus is a fine one.

The bottom line was this: We had a second-story bedroom, and we'd just sprung a gusher. Unless we wanted one less bedroom and a vaulted ceiling on the living room floor, we had to get that mattress out of the house NOW!

Ron, being the engineer that he is, quickly came up with the plan. The layout of our house was such that the stairway led straight down to the front door. I was to open the front door as wide as it could go while he rolled the leaking mattress—still half full of water—out into the upstairs hallway, and then let gravity help roll it down the stairs and out the front door.

Easy as that, right? I mean, who cares that the neighbors

across the street were sitting in lawn chairs on their front porch? Would it matter if they witness a giant waterbed mattress mysteriously rolling out of our house?

Actually, in our neighborhood, probably not.

Still naked, mind you, I safely kept myself behind the front door as I opened it, and then I hid in the playroom off to the side where our kids, who were watching Barney sing his grating *I Love You* song, began to take notice of their mother and the strange situation. *That's right,* I thought to myself as I looked at them both, *Mommy's downstairs naked with the front door wide-open. Don't ask.*

Meanwhile, upstairs, Ron grunted and groaned until the mattress finally rolled out of its frame and landed with a loud *thunk* and *splash* on the floor. What he didn't take into account was the fact that this unframed leaking mattress would become a misshapen slippery amoeba that would take on a life form of its own.

Ron fought it out of our bedroom, and I watched as he struggled to line it up at the top of the stairs. Once he did, he yelled, "Everybody, stand back!" Then he let it go.

Once again, I ducked behind the playroom door for safety.

When it didn't come rolling down the stairs, I poked my head out to see that it was caught up on the banister.

Ron couldn't reach it and said, "You have to come up here and give it a tug."

*You've gotta be kidding me!*

While water sprayed the stairwell in every direction, I mentally debated whether to risk flashing my bare butt to the whole neighborhood.

He yelled, "We're running out of time!"

*He's so dramatic.*

I reluctantly crept out of the playroom, climbed the stairs and gently pulled on the mattress. What I didn't realize was how fast a giant sack of water rolls down a flight of stairs. Also, I didn't realize I'd have no time to make a left turn into the playroom during the descent.

In a split second, I grasped that if I didn't want my cause of death to be listed as "Death by waterbed mattress," I had no choice but to run straight out the front door—screaming and naked—with a waterbed mattress right on my heels. And I did just that.

Once outside, I made an immediate U-turn, ran back into the house and slammed the door. The mattress continued rolling out into the street.

To this day, Ron still tries to convince me that the neighbors were too drunk to understand what they had seen. But, to this day, *I'm* convinced they all pooled their money to buy our house and get us out of the neighborhood.

We might both be right.

# Silence is Golden

by
Petey Fleischmann

My husband (we'll call him "Bill") is a wonderful man. He's funny, sexy, good looking and, well, my idea of a dream man. He also goes out of his way to give me what I want, quoting, "Happy wife, happy life." Still, I sometimes have to trick him to get my way.

A couple of years ago, we decided to get fit by working out several times a week in the pool at the YMCA. After our aqua-aerobics class, Bill and I usually stayed to play in the pool, chasing and splashing and pushing each other into the deep end. In fact, when we first started going to the pool, some of the ladies, noticing how playful we were, asked, "How long have you newlyweds been married?" For the record, we had just celebrated our 23rd anniversary.

Bill always wanted to get out of the pool before I was ready to go. Not having as much body fat as I do, he has a tendency to get cold much more quickly. When he starts to get goose bumps while he's in the water, he also starts to think about all of the projects he wants to do at home and begins urging me to get out of the pool. Since it was a long drive to and from the Y, I preferred to stay as long as possible so that I could burn more calories.

One morning after class, Bill told me he was ready to get out of the water and that he'd meet me at the car. I pleaded with him to stay in the pool for at least another 10 minutes. When 15 minutes had passed, he said, "I'm getting out!" and he headed for the ladder.

Still not ready to go, I caught up with Bill and told him I wanted to talk to him. We moved out of the way of the other people splashing around in the deep end and Bill hung his arm over the pool's edge. I grabbed onto the side with one arm, closed my eyes and whispered some highly erotic things into his ear. Mission accomplished! I knew Bill would NOT leave the pool while his second brain was doing both the thinking AND the pointing! I loved still having so much control over his manhood after all our years together, and I was pleased that I had discovered an ingenious and simple way of keeping him in the pool.

And people think women are the weaker sex! Ha! I felt so powerful, and a completely new world had opened up to me. All I had to do was keep talking dirty, and I'd get what I wanted!

The next day, we attended the usual aqua-aerobics class and played around in the pool afterward, with our usual tomfoolery.

"Too chilly for me," Bill said, "I think I'll get out."

"Just stay a while longer," I pleaded, batting my eyelashes.

"No! Stop that!" he scolded with a grin. "I'm getting out!"

But I had learned exactly how to get my way. I rested my elbow on the edge of the pool, scooted as close to Bill as I could without being obscene then closed my eyes and began to tell him what plans I had for his luscious body as soon as we got home. I was quite specific about what sexy things I would do to him. I listened for a purr. But there was no response . . . no toes sliding up and down my leg . . . no hand on my shoulder . . . no "Petey, behave!" . . . nothing!

Finally, I opened my eyes to see Bill doing a fast crawl stroke to the shallow end. Apparently, he had quietly swum away once I had closed my eyes and started to talk dirty to him, and he hadn't heard a word I'd said. All of my erotic promises had been ignored.

Or had they? I turned my head and saw the man next to me clutching the edge of the pool. His breathing seemed labored, and he had the oddest look on his face, one I've tried to forget, but cannot. He must have thought I was a real pervert . . . and after my graphic descriptions, *he* was probably the man who was too upstanding to leave a spoiled, needy woman in the pool by herself.

I was frozen into stunned silence. My face burned. I'm sure it was crimson. I smiled at the man then swam to the nearby ladder. It was time to go. After all, Bill had already headed for the locker room, and I had many promises to keep once we got home.

# Doing It Where?

by
Kathe Campbell

You are probably aware of the latest recurrent rendering of the *Titanic* movie, where a survivor was interviewed about her affair with a young artist aboard the ship in 1912. Without hesitation, the old woman's response came as a shock to some audiences. "You mean did we do it?" spewed the answer from her 98-year-old lips. Upon hearing her question, my husband, Ken, and I looked at each other and smiled.

Our story wasn't about salt air or an iceberg seizing a huge ocean liner. It was about my man's race for home, driving hell-bent, afire with frenzied fury to hold, touch and eagerly embrace his "joy."

I wish I could say it was that six o'clock ritual that turns hot-and-heavy newlyweds into suck-faced idiots, all the while supper incinerates on the stove.

The passion was about being laid all right, except it

wasn't I who was getting laid. It was cedar strips. Laid over our canoe's building jig, the cedar strips were heated, bent, shaped, glued and clamped a thousand times. Eager to get the evening show on the road, Ken could barely choke down dinner or squeeze out a little peck on the cheek. My job was artfully aesthetic for the most part—measuring parts, ribbing, working on benches, mixing glue and sanding, sanding, sanding. Oh, that cedar, a lovely fragrance that God forgot to empower with a soul. Or did He?

It was about the telling repeatedly of a young lad's summer adventures, paddling a leaky old wreck up and down the ever-menacing Columbia River. Then the wait until layers of transparent fiberglass and epoxy coating inside and out dried. Days slid by until I could show off my perfectly painted lettering that read, "DELIVERANCE." I wondered how many of those monikers would show up on canoe bows after that chiller movie.

Launching our beauty onto serene waters, we paddled out onto a desolate, pitch-black lake just a stone's throw from the Hemingway digs near Sun Valley, Idaho. I can still hear the soothing sound of ripples lapping against the sides of our handcrafted vessel.

Our Hollywood-worthy story is about Deliverance's christening. Building her was just foreplay. His Majesty spent the first hour of her maiden voyage convincing me that there are a number of devices that increase sexual arousal, particularly in women. Chief among them was diamond-studded trinkets, a Mercedes-Benz, or, in this case, making whoopee in our lovely new canoe.

Did we do it? Oh, yes! There must be a certain area of the brain that controls those "four F's"—feeling, fumbling, floundering and, uh, "mating." I'm too much of a lady to use that last word.

It seemed rather interesting that our watery rocking and rolling sounded just like great sex. I suppose it didn't matter how or where we did it, so long as we hadn't sprung any leaks or frightened the fish. Yep, it was a funky way to baptize a canoe, not to mention celebrating a different kind of blessed event exactly nine months later.

Today, Deliverance hangs upside down in the rafters of our donkey barn. We migrated to a Montana mountain to homestead in God's wilderness nowhere near a lake. Bath towels folded neatly over her paddles, we settled in our log home to celebrate 53 years of wedded passions. Regular treks to the barn bring an impish grin to my face. "Keep up those F's, girl."

# Our First Time

by
Belinda Cohen

OK, so we did it in the outdoor hot tub. It seemed like a good idea at the time. A 6-foot privacy fence surrounded our backyard. The children were gone for at least two hours.

We climbed into the bubbling, steaming water for that ever-special first time. Not *that* first time, but the first time in our new hot tub. And yes, it was all we hoped for and more. Afterward, I cuddled my cheek against my husband's chest and gazed up at the stars. "Why don't we do this more often?"

He wholeheartedly agreed. Every Sunday, while the kids were at church, would be our official date night. Praise the Lord.

With our magical evening coming to an end, Hubby grabbed his trunks and slid them back on. "I'll pick up the kids," he offered.

Amazing how agreeable husbands can be after a raucous encounter in the hot tub. I snatched my top out of the bubbling, churning water and fastened it around my back. He helped me tie the top part around my neck.

"Do you see the bottoms?" I asked.

My husband and I looked like the Coast Guard on a rescue mission, straining our vision and swishing through the swirling swells to locate the bikini bottoms.

"I need more light," my husband said. He returned with two flashlights. We held them high above the water like helicopter search beams.

"Found them," he said, pointing to the bunched up fabric wedged in the bottom of the return valve. I plunged my hand deep into the water and tugged. They refused to budge.

My husband killed the power to the motor, hoping to relieve pressure on the valve. It was no use—they weren't going anywhere.

"You'll need to call a plumber," he told me with a straight face.

"No way!" I looked at him like he was crazy. "I'm not calling a plumber to fish out my bikini bottoms from the hot tub."

I rubbed my chin. There must be a better solution. We're adults. We're educated. We could figure this out.

Tuesday morning, Gus's Plumbing pulled into the driveway. His business slogan blazed across the side of his truck, "If it don't flush, don't cuss, call Gus." I happily sighed. This wasn't going to be embarrassing at all.

Gus hopped out of the truck and emptied a wad of tobacco from his cheek onto the grass. I looked away and pretended not to be disgusted.

I explained to Gus, "Someone accidentally dropped an article of clothing into the hot tub."

"What kinda clothing are we talking about?" He cocked his head to the side.

"A bathing suit," I said, refusing to avert my gaze.

Gus flashed me a lascivious grin that exposed the residual chewing tobacco between his front teeth. I sat in the shade while he worked his plumber magic on the hot tub. I spent the next 15 minutes trying to look at anything except the predictable butt crack peeking over the top of Gus's work belt.

Finally, he emerged victorious. He held my teal bikini bottoms above his head like a trophy. "This what you're lookin' for?"

"Yes, thanks. How much do I owe you?"

Gus laughed. "I oughta do it for free. It'll be worth it to tell my buddies about this one."

"Gus, we're all adults here. Can you just write up the invoice so I can make out a check?" I was growing impatient with his innuendo.

"Ewww weee girl. You musta had one heluva party in that Jacuzzi. I mean, with that fiery attitude you got there, and all."

With that thought in mind, we effectively ended any possibility of additional romance in the hot tub. Hubby and I are strictly a dinner-and-a-movie couple these days. And it's going to stay that way.

# Entertaining Your Fantasies

The naked truth!

# Pink Roses

by
Jan Stephens

One gorgeous fall day, I was driving home—alone—on winding roads lined with trees of every shade of gold and red. I emphasize "alone" because, on such a lovely drive, nobody should be alone. But, I'd been divorced for eight months. Although I'd been enjoying an online correspondence with someone I liked very much, we hadn't yet met, and would not until the following month when I'd relocate to Dallas.

And so, feeling rather lonely on that cool, crisp Saturday evening, I watched the sun set and tried to distract myself by reveling in the matchless golden light autumn cast upon everything.

I decided it was a perfect evening for a bottle of wine and a nice steak and stopped at the grocery store on the way home. Pushing my cart toward the meat department, I passed a lovely bouquet of pink roses. I stopped and turned back to the flowers, stood there and briefly recollected roses I'd been given in the past as I pressed my nose into the soft, pink petals and sniffed. Feeling a little maudlin, I wondered if anyone would ever give me roses again. Then, my "put-on-your-big-girl-panties" voice spoke up: *Oh, stop that. Just buy the darned roses for yourself!*

I snickered. *Buy them for myself?* I answered myself in my head. *Why not?*

And so, I did. And they changed my life.

Back in the car heading home, my "that-was-a-silly-thing-to-do" voice barged in: *You bought roses for yourself? Now, what did you do to deserve that? You'd better come up with a pretty good story about how you got them.*

So, being a writer, I concocted this story, all the while grinning at my naughtiness.

### 

It was Bikes, Blues & Barbecue weekend, and I felt lonely watching motorcycle after motorcycle pass by. I wanted to be that woman on the back seat, pressed against her partner's body, the bike rumbling between her legs. Add to that a beautiful fall day . . . well, you get the picture.

I decided to stop at the grocery store and pick up a few things. As I was leaving, I passed a convoy of bikers gathered at the outskirts of the lot.

Something made me turn my car around to go talk to them. Usually, I'm pretty shy, but my longing was deep.

I pulled up next to them, got out of my car and blurted,

"Hi, my name's Jan. Anyone want to give me a ride?"

Seven burly men stared at me as if unsure I was serious. The four women crossed their arms and glared. Then a guy in leathers stepped forward and pointed to a shiny, black Harley. "Sure. Hop on," he said.

He seemed nice enough—and alone—so I did. I was nervous, but also excited, in every sense of the word. I mounted the bike and searched for a place to put my hands. But alas, there was no place, except around his waist.

When he revved the engine and took off, I was surprised at the power I felt between my legs and unsure of what was vibrating through my body—the bike or the desire. Let's see. A bike rumbling between my legs or my body pressed against a handsome stranger. It was the latter.

I kept telling myself I was crazy, but the ride was glorious.

After about 20 minutes, we rolled into the grocery store parking lot. I felt a warm buzz, and without thinking, I asked, "Would you like me to give *you* a ride now?"

Oh, yes, those naughty words did come from my mouth, but at least I asked nicely. It was almost primal. I couldn't control it.

His bike buddies practically backed away and gawked at him, as if thinking, "What are you gonna do now, buddy?"

I'm pretty sure the red I saw across his face was not the light of the setting sun.

He smiled, almost shyly, and replied, "Well, hop on again." Then, as if to protect my honor, he whispered into my ear, "You sure about this? My hotel is just down the road."

Well, of course I wasn't sure. But, in a split second, I

convinced myself I'd feel too guilty if I offered then chickened out. So, I mounted his bike once again.

That was all the answer he needed, and we roared out of the lot together.

I can't tell you what the hotel room looked like or how we got into bed—I was on autopilot. All I know is, the sex was hard and fast, just what I needed.

Afterward, he held me for a little while, told me his name was "Joe." He took just enough time, gave me just enough tenderness that I didn't feel used.

When he returned me to the grocery store, he asked me to wait while he ran in for something.

He returned with a bouquet of the most beautiful pink roses I'd ever seen. "Thank you kindly, Jan," he said.

And then we went our separate ways.

### 

So how did those pink roses change my life?

Well, remember my online correspondence? The man I liked very much? His name was Steve, and as I began my nightly email to him, I pondered about whether to tell him the real story about how the pink roses came into my possession—or the one I had made up.

Just then, I morphed into the daring heroine from my biker story. Actually, I didn't change into her. Instead, I lifted a veil, because that mischievous, sexual woman had always been a part of me, buried deep beneath a shroud of "should be."

I started my email by telling Steve I'd been feeling a little lonely that night, and then sent him my story, as if it had really happened. My "that-was-a-silly-thing-to-do" voice started screaming: *I can't believe you hit the 'send' button!*

But the bigger part of me was glad I had. Later that night, Steve and I talked for hours about my email, our love of writing and our attempts to be what others expect us to be. And last, but certainly not least, we talked about our attitudes about sex. Our veils of "should be" had been lifted.

Steve now knows every part of who I am. The naughty and the nice.

You might ask which he likes more, but a good girl doesn't tell all her secrets.

# The Standing O

by
Dahlynn McKowen

There is a running joke between my husband, Ken, and me, having to do with a "Standing O." Of course, the "O" is for "orgasm." And it doesn't mean having an orgasm while standing—even though that's fun—but rather that I'm ready for action whenever he is.

I like sex. No, I *love* sex and can never seem to get enough. One rainy day, I challenged my hubby to see how many times he could get it up in a 24-hour period. Ken rose to my challenge, and after making love to me seven times in less than 16 hours, I extended a white flag. I had had enough.

Years later, we found ourselves on a writing assignment, exploring upstate New York and Massachusetts during the month of October. The two-week trip was eventful and busy as we traipsed through the Adirondacks, visited famed Civil War sites and took hundreds of fall-color photos. We also visited the homes of famous Massachusetts authors, from *Moby Dick*'s Herman Melville's house in Pittsfield to Louisa May Alcott's Orchard House in Concord, the setting for her novel *Little Women*. We painted Boston red, visiting all the historic monuments and JKF's presidential museum. We then traveled south to the United First Parish Church in Quincy, where both President John Adams and President John Quincy Adams are interred.

It was late on day 10 of our trip when we arrived in Plymouth, the home of the Pilgrim landing. Finding our hotel, we ordered in pizza then popped open a few beers.

Our room was one of two in a duplex setup, separate from the main three-story hotel. Being a single-story unit, we were thrilled that there was no one above us. I saw our neighbors arrive when paying the pizza delivery guy—if I had to guess, our fellow duplex dwellers were in their early 60s, just like Ken, who is 13 years my senior. I said hello to them before closing the door. The man smiled and nodded, but the woman ignored me.

As we ate, Ken and I planned our itinerary for the next day, hoping to get out to Cape Cod if time permitted. Exhausted after a long day of running from place to place, we collapsed into bed. Fooling around wasn't even on our minds.

The next morning, our planned itinerary took us to tourist spots like Plymouth Rock and the reconstructed Mayflower. We also explored the town's cemeteries, including Burial Hill, with plots of famed Pilgrims such as governor William Bradford.

Around 2 P.M., the weather turned. The wind kicked up,

and the rain started to fall in sheets. There would be no Cape Cod trip that day. On the way back to our hotel, we bought canned soup to heat up in the microwave, along with cheese, crackers and a bottle of wine.

Back at the hotel, Ken asked me what we should do with the rest of our day since we were stuck inside. Of course, we both knew the answer.

"What do you think?" I teased.

"Well, we could try to break my record of seven times," Ken said, a grin slowly growing across his face and a hard-on slowly growing inside his pants.

"We can't do that. What if the neighbors hear us?"

"Last night, we didn't even hear a peep from them, not even the TV set," Ken answered. "I bet the walls are thick since it gets so cold here."

"Game on. Let me take a bubble bath first," I said, heading into the bathroom. "We can go a few rounds then have dinner."

For Ken to break his record, he would have had to get an erection eight times between the hours of 5 P.M. and bedtime, which, we both knew, wasn't going to happen. No all-nighter for me, as this girl needed her beauty sleep before a full day of sightseeing on Cape Cod. But we made the most of our time together, along with lots of noise, which, hopefully, drowned out by the nasty weather. By 11, I was more than satisfied and pleaded to my stud to go to sleep.

The storm passed that night, and the sun shone brilliantly the next morning. Ken and I got ready quickly then loaded our photo gear and backpacks into our rental car for the trip to the Cape Cod National Seashore.

While taking one of many trips to the car, I noticed our neighbors. They were sitting outside their door at a small table, drinking coffee. As I had the night before, I offered a greeting. The man smiled, the woman glared.

"What's wrong with her?" I asked Ken when I went back inside our room. "She won't even acknowledge me."

"I don't know. Maybe she's not a friendly person," Ken said as he checked the room to make sure we hadn't forgotten anything.

"OK, *you* say hello to her when you go out there and see if she talks to you," I said.

Closing the door and making sure it was locked, Ken turned to say hello. But before he could, the man rose from his seat and began clapping, slowly at first then faster and faster. In absolute disgust, the woman jumped up from her chair and ran into their hotel room.

"Ah, thanks, I guess," Ken said to the man, who had reached out to shake Ken's hand.

The lesson learned that day was to never assume anything, unless you're guaranteed a standing O.

# Cinderella and the Codpiece

by
Rosie Sorenson

By the time I turned 49, I'd had sex with more men than the number of casseroles my mother had baked for our Lutheran church potlucks.

Lusting with Carl—the Tesla of sex machines—could have powered the globe 17 times over during our yearlong romance. Except for his teensy bit of narcissism, which was easy to overlook when I was under him, I might still be at his side. But, damn it, when he left me out of his Christmas plans, his value tumbled faster than I could say, "WTF?"

After I dumped him, I slept for six days, feeling more like the dumpee than the dumper, afraid I'd be alone the rest of my life. But on the seventh day, I woke up to the realization that being single wasn't the worst that could happen. No! I'd already done the worst thing by putting up with and putting out for men who were as wrong for me as a string bikini.

Soon after I kicked Carl to the curb, I did what I always do when I'm in pain. I ate seven squares of dark chocolate (70-percent cacao) and surfed the Internet. I developed a sudden interest in Cinderella. To my amazement, I learned that she was born in ninth-century China. This no doubt explains the foot-fetish thing, what with the tiny slipper and all. Now headquartered at Disneyland, this blood-sucking tick has infected the entire civilized world—especially the souls of women—with the notion that if we're only nice enough, patient enough and pretty enough, we will be rewarded with a wonderful man who will take good care of us forever.

*Right.*

It seemed obvious to me that the fairytale had less to do with Cinderella than it did with Prince Charming and his sense of entitlement. He was entitled to have women mutilate themselves for a chance to receive his hand in marriage. Remember those two ugly stepsisters and their attempts to cut off their heels and toes so they could shove their size 11s into the precious size-4 slippers? You can't get more entitled than that.

But what of the other Cinderella story, the one that hasn't yet surfaced?

In this as-yet-to-be-discovered tale, Prince Charming is just an ordinary working-class guy named "Ralph" who happens to wangle an invitation to the Grand Ball given by Cinderella, the fairest and most wealthy princess in the land. She has let it be known that she is available to dance the dance of mating.

During the evening's festivities, after waltzing with our handsome Ralph, Cinderella falls in love and lust. However, just before midnight, our Ralphie disappears. Fleeing the castle grounds, he notices too late that he's lost his codpiece (a leather pouch into which a gentleman inserts his manhood). *Oh well, can't turn back now,* he says to himself. His golden coach has already begun reverting to its original form of a kumquat.

Cinderella is distraught. Upon finding his codpiece on the ballroom floor, she dispatches her minions to scour the countryside to locate the man who captured her heart and whose "member" fit neatly into the pouch.

All the prince-wannabes are so eager for a chance to be chosen by the princess that they attempt to fool the minions. The more amply endowed men whack off a few inches, believing they might then be able to squeeze into the goatskin pouch. Their underendowed brothers resort to strapping sausages onto their organs to ensure a snug fit. Alas, one by one, they are found to be frauds.

The search widens, and finally, the party of minions arrives at the orchard where our lowly Ralph perches high in a peach tree, picking fruit for his master. The master tells the minions, "You needn't bother with old Ralphie here. He couldn't possibly be the one you seek."

The minions reply, "Oh, no sir, we must check every member in the land. Our lady has so decreed." The master, not wanting to lose his head or anything, reluctantly calls out to Ralph, "Hey boy, come down here posthaste, they want to look you over." Upon hearing this, Ralph smooths back his hair.

Ralph slowly descends the ladder and faces the minions. They hand him the codpiece and watch, astonished, as he slips into it. A perfect fit. "Voila! The prince has been found!"

Ralph is whisked away forthwith to Cinderella in a golden coach, and they are married in a lavish non-denominational ceremony. No more peach picking for our dear Ralphie.

On their wedding night, the lovely Cinderella asks no more of Prince Ralph than that he be faithful, submissive and beautiful forever, and that he satisfy her every sexual desire while, at the same time, of course, showering her with dark chocolate!

*If only.*

# Salon Tales

by
Molly O'Connor

Elizabeth was a tall, slim redhead with regal bearing and a decidedly elegant British accent. One could imagine her seated on a roan horse and picture her as an English baroness about to gallop off on her handsome steed.

She was a new client, and I had yet to develop a rapport with her. So, as I did with all new clients, I initiated the conversation by talking about the weather and a current event happening in our small town.

I ran my fingers through her freshly washed hair, lifting the strands and letting them fall into place. "Can I make a suggestion? I would like to accent your natural curl, take away the bulk and razor cut it so it is easy to manage." I was talking to her image through the mirror of my downtown hair salon.

"My dear, you can do whatever you want as long as

Charles immediately drags me off to the bedroom and ravishes me."

My eyes became the size of saucers—hers were twinkling.

"Charles is my husband, darling. Sex is what has kept our marriage fresh and exciting for 15 years."

That set the tone for our years as client and hairdresser. Elizabeth became one of my favorite clients, and I selfishly booked her appointments on a regular basis as my last customer of the week. I always closed the salon for the weekend with a smile on my face. Her zest for life and sex produced story after story. Her formal English accent always seemed a contradiction to her recounting of personal tidbits about life and love with "Chah-les."

I later met Charles—he, too, was the picture of elegance. He was straight-backed with a chiseled nose and high cheekbones that would have any lusting gal panting.

"Charles and I are off to Florida for a wee bit of a holiday without the girls. I simply have to tell you, our two daughters—one is 11, the other 12—have a lot to learn about sexual appetites."

"Oh, really?"

"I inadvertently overheard them talking about their father and me. I was walking along the upstairs hallway when I heard the younger one ask her sister if she thought Charles and I did *it*. I have to admit, I silently backed against the wall with my ear to their open bedroom door when I heard this. You won't believe what they decided."

"What?" I was leaning forward so as not to miss a word.

"My older, wiser daughter announced with authority that it was obvious that Mommy and Daddy had only done *it* twice because there were just two of them. I almost dropped the laundry basket."

After the laughter and knowing looks subsided, there was a definite lull in the conversation.

"So where are you going in Florida?"

"We've rented a lovely apartment in Fort Myers. It's the second time we've been there."

I sensed a story.

"The last time we went was years ago; we left the girls with friends and his mother went with us. In fact, if truth be known, she treated us to that holiday."

"Lucky you!"

"We had a lovely two-bedroom suite overlooking the ocean. Mommy had the smaller room, and we had the larger one with a balcony. The weather was perfect—in the mid-80s—but we had a wee bit of a problem. The air conditioner was broken, and the suite was beastly warm. Charles and I were quite comfortable because the double doors to the balcony let in soft sea breezes. Mother's room was ghastly hot, so she decided to drag her mattress onto the balcony so she, too, could enjoy the cool night air. This left Charles and me absolutely no privacy and our hormonal urges were raging. We are not quiet lovers, so the situation was awkward, if not totally impossible."

"Oh, Elizabeth, whatever did you do?"

"As bedtime approached, Charles suggested a walk on the beach to watch the moon rise. Mother, thank goodness, begged off, as was our hope. Armed with a blanket and a bottle of wine, we headed for a secluded alcove and relished the romantic setting—envisioning a dip in the ocean, licking the salt off each other's bodies, watching the moon rise, racing along the beach—all creating the scene for perfect lovemaking."

She stopped talking. I held the hairbrush, immobilized in midair.

"And?"

"Well, my dear, at 20, sex on the beach is very romantic—at 40, its damned sandy!"

Hoots of laughter filled the salon, as, by this time, everyone was tuned in. Not all her tales were gritty (my pun), but nearly always ended with a lusty romp between the sheets.

Prepping Elizabeth for a New Year's celebration, I asked how her Christmas had been.

"Lovely dear, perfectly lovely. We went to the Christmas Eve candlelight church service and since the evening was so beautiful with the gently falling snow, we walked to and from church. It's our custom to have a light snack and open our parcels after church on Christmas Eve. Charles gave me a lovely pair of pearl earrings, and I gave him a lovely handknit sweater.

After the gifts, the children were tucked in, and I went to turn down the lights. Charles said he was so taken with his sweater that he wanted to try it on immediately. When I got to our bedroom, there he was clad in only his sweater with his frontal-piece standing at full attention like a soldier ready for duty. This outrageous sight took me unaware, and

I burst into laughter, so giddy that I couldn't stop. Tears were running down my cheeks, and before I knew it, Charles was laughing, too—the soldier fell before combat, and we rolled into bed, holding our sore sides."

"Now, Elizabeth, that can't be how your story ends."

"Well, my dear, when Rome fell, it did rise again."

I lost touch with Elizabeth and Charles when I sold my salon. They have to be in their 80s by now, and I still picture them cuddled under the blankets, sharing a warm embrace and enjoying each other's caresses. They will have aged, but I'm sure their lust remains young and vigorous.

# Peeping Toms

by

Stephen Hayes

Writing coaches caution anyone from starting a story with, "It was a dark and stormy night." But I've always wanted to begin a tale with these words—and now you know what I think of writing coaches.

Anyway, my wife and I had only been married a few years and were living in a duplex in Oxnard, California, so close to the beach that our driveway was covered in sand. One stormy evening, my wife phoned to say she was leaving work late and was in no mood to fix dinner. "I'll pick up something on the way home," she said.

I felt guilty that she was the one caught in the storm. "It's raining pretty hard. Be careful," I said, just as the electricity went out.

While waiting in the darkness for her to arrive home, I lifted a blind and glanced out our front window to check on the storm. Without street lamps, I couldn't see much, but I could hear the wind howling like a banshee in heat, along with the sound of swirling sand scratching the world raw.

A light winked on across the street, the golden glow of an oil lamp. I could clearly see into the bedroom of the young couple who'd recently rented that bungalow. I'd yet to speak with them; for some reason, I'd been put off by their attractiveness and athleticism. They stood beside a large bed. He leaned toward her, bent down and kissed her long and hard. She unbuckled his jeans.

It felt wrong to be ogling them as they undressed, their perfect bodies reflected in the circular mirror of an old vanity hugging a wall. I considered lowering the blind but couldn't. It was like watching a porn movie being filmed before my very eyes. What if they needed extras?

As the wind whipped sand around the edges of their window, I watched as they pleasured each other. I'd been married a few years to a woman with a healthy sexual appetite, and I'd read *Everything You Always Wanted to Know About Sex, but Were Afraid to Ask,* not to mention my familiarity with *Kama Sutra*, whose illustrations I'd committed to memory. I wasn't without a certain expertise in this area and considered myself a competent swordsman, but the Olympian acrobatics and exuberant gymnastics of this energetic couple were far beyond anything I'd imagined, much less attempted. Whereas I'd be huffing and puffing, with sweat dripping from me in unsightly fashion, this couple was clearly not out of breath. Instead of sweating like railroad workers shoveling coal into a blazing furnace, their naked bodies glowed like burnished gold in the lamplight.

I lost track of time, the window steaming over from my hard breathing. A noise alerted me to the fact that I wasn't alone. My wife was standing behind me, a boxed pizza in her hands. I could feel my face turn scarlet, and I wondered what she was thinking. *I've married a voyeur, a Peeping Tom!*

But her eyes weren't on me—she was watching the couple across the street, the marathon pair into their second hour of lovemaking. I took the pizza from her hands and went to the kitchen. When I returned, she was still standing there, watching as intently as I had been. I tried to remove her coat, but she was transfixed by the show and wouldn't budge.

If she was going to enjoy the performance, I saw no reason I shouldn't, as well. At that moment, we witnessed something taking place in the bedroom across the street that shocked both of us. I couldn't believe what I was seeing, and neither could my wife, whose jaw was hanging as low as mine was.

My wife finally tore her eyes from the window. She swung her purse at me, yelling, "You told me that was IM-POSSIBLE!"

She stomped off.

Back in the bungalow, the dude who'd made me feel like an incompetent kindergartener was no longer naked. He and his lady had donned terry robes, and they were now waving at me.

# The Golf Lesson

by
Darcy Tarbell

I was behaving like a pimple-faced, sexually distracted adolescent suffering from unrequited lust. At the age of 35, I was weaving sexual fantasies in full Technicolor—starring me, of course—and a handsome, charming and maddeningly aloof co-worker. The action started the moment I got a whiff of his aftershave each morning as he strolled by my desk. Unfortunately, I was employed in the banking industry, not the film industry.

"You have to find something in common with him," a friend advised. "You need a prelude to your dive between the sheets. You said he's always talking about golf."

Golf was a brilliant suggestion. I'd watched a few tournaments on TV. I noticed that the players never sweat. Besides, golf looked effortless. How difficult could it be? I scheduled my first lesson.

After meeting my female instructor at the golf shop, we headed to the practice range. The pro instructed me to position my feet parallel to the tee. "Swing the club back and let the weight of the club head do the work for you. Just follow through to complete your swing."

I chopped hard, powering my shot toward the 185-yard marker. Or so I thought. I looked down. The ball remained precisely where it had been placed.

Golf was proving harder than I had imagined.

After hitting 50-odd balls, I'd successfully driven fewer than 15 of them off the tee, none more than 35 yards. Wanting to be supportive, the pro said, "There's an adage, 'Drive for show, putt for dough.'"

As we moved to the putting green, I was confident that this part of the game would be easier for me. All I had to do was get a little ball into the hole.

She placed six balls at various distances from the hole. She effortlessly sunk each one as she casually walked around the green. "Now it's your turn. Just remember to follow through," she said.

*And let the club head do the work*, I repeated to myself as I took a full swing of the club.

"Airborne!" I yelled, the ball popping 25 feet straight up.

"Fore! The correct term is 'fore,'" the pro said. I thought I detected a hint of exasperation in her voice.

After an inordinate amount of time, the lesson ended. "You're a natural at this game," she said. "Maybe we could get together sometime," she added suggestively.

I knew she was being generous in her assessment of my attempt at golf. As flattered as I was, I had cast a different lead in my sexual fantasy. I declined her invitation.

But my encounter with the golf pro made for a good

weekend story. So engaging was I Monday morning that my handsome co-worker, the one I was lusting after, offered to help me with the missing elements of my game.

"All you'll need is your pitching wedge," he said when he called to arrange a time. "Meet me at the practice range, near the putting green."

That day, I chose my most sheer lace bra and pantie set. Never mind that the brassiere offered no support and was made of cheap red nylon, stiffened into shape with fabric finish. I adjusted the skimpy undergarment over my ample chest. I wanted to look sultry and sexy under my golf gear. I was more concerned with making my fantasies a reality than perfecting my golf game.

Before I arrived at the golf course, my co-worker had purchased a large bucket containing 100 practice balls and had settled in next to an elevated green. He chipped the ball into the air, and it landed with a plop then slowly rolled toward the hole. He held his club softly in his right hand and executed a short, gentle swing. Over and over, he repeated his stroke with precision, while I stood by appreciatively. He was good. I felt my face flush with excitement, imagining how good he was elsewhere.

"It's your turn," he said.

I stepped up to the pile of balls. I held my club softly in my right hand and straightened my arms out away from my body, resting the club head next to a ball.

"No, no, no. You need to step in closer," he said.

I stepped forward, swung and missed the ball.

"No! You're doing it all wrong!" he said, repeating his instructions and adding, "Keep your head DOWN."

I could feel the sweat bead up on my forehead. My next 10

attempts were not much better, although I did manage to rocket one ball onto the first tee box.

He kept repeating the same phrases, each time speaking more slowly and loudly. Perhaps he thought I no longer spoke English. Then he muttered under his breath, "You swing like a fat man." I knew what he was talking about—men who hold their arms out over their bellies. It throws their balance off. I needed to swing my arms through my breasts, rather than over them. I tried it. The ball popped up and skidded across the green.

"Excellent," he said, his attitude changing.

Confident of his ability to impart knowledge, he proceeded to school my every shot. I just focused on pushing my arms through my boobs. Because I was wearing my "why-pay-good-money-for-clothing-that-is-going-to-end-up-on-the-floor" lingerie set, I was in agony. It was like sanding my nipples off with a Brillo pad.

I chipped my way through that entire bucket of balls. Sweat slid down the back of my knees and pooled in my shoes. My neck ached from holding my head down. Blisters appeared on my hand. All I wanted to do was rip my clothes off and take a cool shower. It seemed my co-worker had a similar idea. His libido had been peaked by the pheromones I was exuding. But my exertion combined with perspiration had extinguished my passion.

Later that evening, with the bra in the trash, I knew my fantasy had succumbed to reality. I was willing to let it go. But I was not prepared to give up my fat-man swing.

# CHAPTER TEN

# Kick Him to the Curb

Don't stub your toe.

# Goofballitis

by
Karen Gaebelein

I've been on many dates. I don't want to estimate how many because that would only make me feel old—something I try to avoid at all costs.

I must be afflicted with a sickness that causes me to attract unusual men. The medical community has not yet recognized this malady. So until they do, I refer to my sickness as "goofballitis."

Let me explain. When I first meet men, they seem normal. But after a while, they become "goofballs." Goofballitis—with "G.B." being the acronym for such men—has given me the unique experience of meeting guys who do or say things beyond ridiculous.

For example, one G.B. arrived at my door wearing a scuba suit underneath his clothes. The reason? He liked the feel of rubber against his skin. I never let this one past my doorway, and when I asked him to leave, I gave him my rubber doormat as a souvenir.

Another G.B. asked me out for a cup of coffee and wondered if I would be opposed to slapping him with the leather whip he had in his car. This was after choir practice. A friend of mine had fixed us up—she thought he was a nice, quiet, good guy. Ha! That's a big, "No, I don't think so!"

When yet another G.B. asked me if I would be opposed to inserting an electrical appliance, most often thought of for the pleasure of women, in various places on both of us, I immediately excused myself. From another room, I called my friend. As a repressed Catholic, I wanted to check with her to see if this was the new normal. And, if so, when had "normal" changed? And could she explain it to me? I also asked her, "Should I call 911 if the appliance gets stuck in one of the specified areas?"

When she couldn't stop laughing, I hung up. Returning to the bedroom, I explained to the G.B. that I was a low-mileage Catholic girl and that he was a little too advanced for my taste. I sent him packing.

You may be thinking, "Girl, where do you hang out? Porno shops? And do you have sex with everyone you date?" Again, my answer is "No."

I am old school. I believe in romance. I fondly remember the fireworks that went off in my head when I had my first kiss. And how my knees turned to JELL-O when I was kissed by someone I cared about, that first tender moment with someone I loved. I remember the heat I felt from his hand when mine brushed against it. That's what I am talking about! Good times! Passion!

The truth is that I met these G.B.s at church functions and through dating websites that promote matching people who are like-minded. Perhaps checking *fishing* as a hobby on the dating profile put me into the category of men who prefer wetsuits to jockeys. I checked an interest in *technology*, too. Was that how I got the "appliance" guy?

At this stage of my life, I have taken a break from dating and the ultimate dance of shake, rattle and roll. One day, I will bump into a guy who strikes my fancy. And as long as I can find my fancy and it still works, we should both have a good time.

# Ménage à Twerp

by
Marsha Wight Wise

Back in my B.J. days (before John, my husband . . . what did you think I meant?), I had a thing for Jewish boys. I don't know why I was drawn to them like Kim Kardashian to a plastic-surgeon convention, but I was. Given a man with a prominent nose and a last name ending in –man, –stein or –berg, I immediately pictured myself under the huppah . . . the Jewish wedding canopy.

So the day I went to my local pharmacy and discovered they had hired a good-looking, albeit short, new pharmacist named Mitch Goldman, I was in my element. I was already calculating how many questions I could get away with asking him at the counter before the store would start charging me for advice.

The good news is I wasn't arrested for stalking because Mitch also took a liking to me. Being only 4 feet 11 inches tall, I've always appealed to shorter guys . . . and my blond hair, cute tochus, and DD cup size didn't hurt, either. When I dropped off my prescription for allergy meds, Mitch said he would call me when it was ready. And he did. That's when our tumultuous romance began.

After our first date, Mitch didn't call me for a week. For months, I bought every lame excuse he gave as to why I would not hear from him after our dates. And if I did question him, he would always turn it around on me and ask why *I* was trying to make *him* feel bad.

Then I finally came to my senses. At a time when we hadn't seen much of each other, I finally decided I needed to let Mitch go. But then, a bootie-call from him caught me in a particularly vulnerable mood. Against my better judgment, I allowed him to reel me back in.

When I arrived at his place that night, I wasn't the only one to receive a call from Mitch. Sitting on the sofa was a pretty Asian-American girl whose face reflected the same confusion I felt. As soon as he introduced us, she began to make excuses that she needed to leave. But Mitch assured her she should stay.

The three of us made awkward chitchat, and then Mitch offered us drinks. When he left the room, she asked me, "Did you know he called me, too?"

"No," I answered.

She grabbed her belongings and quickly left.

Mitch came running when he heard the door slam. He sealed his fate by saying, "What did you say to make her leave?"

I was livid, not only about that comment but also about

all the times I had allowed him to treat me like a schlock.

Mitch insisted I go after her, and I did, but not for the reasons he thought. I caught up with her at her car and learned from her that she had just met him. With that, I gave her the lowdown on what to expect in a relationship with Mitch. We both agreed that our boy was looking for a three-some, and we shared a laugh. She left, vowing never again to take his call. I said I was done with him, too. And I meant it.

Deciding to head home rather than return to Mitch's apartment, I lay awake all night. I was beyond pissed and decided that the best revenge would be to get even.

By dawn, I had a plan. I called my BFF Veronica and ran my idea by her. She was ecstatic to help and happy that I had finally seen the light when it came to Mitch. But I needed one more person for the plan to work. Veronica called back and said her friend Michelle was in.

I called Mitch and apologized for having thwarted his ménage à trois. Then I asked, "How could I possibly make it up to you?"

True to his narcissism, Mitch said, "I'm sure you have a friend who would be up for it." He had played right into my hands.

A few days later, I called Mitch and told him I had a friend—Michelle—who was always game for a good, raunchy time and had agreed to meet him at my place. I'm certain I heard the zipper of his Dockers groan with the sudden increase of pressure from within. In the nine months I had known Mitch, I had learned never to mention his height or that I was sure that, at age 25, he was still shopping in the junior's department at Sears.

I smiled over the fact that I was about to pierce his Achilles' heel.

Veronica and Michelle arrived at my place early. We rehearsed the script and reviewed our positions in the room. Since Mitch knew Veronica, she couldn't be visible. Thus, she was our safety net in case things got out of hand. She took her position behind the basement door, just off the living room, cordless phone in hand and finger poised to dial 911.

Michelle was so eager to play her role that she had dressed like a $20 hooker—sheer black lace blouse, no bra and tight black pants. I had on a bodysuit that displayed my fabulous DDs. I knew Mitch wouldn't be able to walk upright less than 10 seconds after crossing the threshold.

He showed up, grinning as if he had just won the lottery. It was obvious he liked what he saw. He and I settled onto the sofa with Michelle sitting in a chair across from us. After small talk, our eager beaver dove right into the subject at hand—or at least it would be in his hand later that night.

"So, Michelle—Marsha tells me you like threesomes?"

Blushing, Michelle said, "I've only had one with my old boyfriend, but I really liked it. When Marsha called, I thought, 'Why not'?"

By this point, Mitch was so excited he rubbed his sweating palms on his pant legs. "What's your favorite part?" he asked Michelle.

"Seeing my boyfriend's face as we pleasured him." She had obviously read too many Harlequin romances to come up with that line.

"Why don't you sit over here with us?" Mitch said, patting the sofa.

Michelle sat beside him, snuggled in close and none too shyly placed her hand on his bulging manhood, giving it a playful squeeze. He groaned and rolled his head back.

Then Michelle delivered the line we had practiced. Jumping up, she said to me, "Marsha, I'm sorry. I can't do this! I came here to be with a man and he's . . . he's . . . he's the size of a 14-year-old boy!" On cue, she grabbed her jacket and purse then left.

If only this had been during the Smartphone age, I would have a photo to share with you. To say Mitch was mad would be like saying the Duggars have just a few kids. Smoke drifted from his ears, and he couldn't form a complete sentence. "What the f_ _k just . . . what a see-you-next-Tuesday (edited because I'm a lady) . . . she didn't . . . what . . . didn't . . . I . . . I . . . I have to go NOW!"

I remained in character and tried to soothe Mitch, but he stormed out.

That very night, I regained my confidence. I also understood, for the first time, the meaning of closure. No more toxic, co-dependent relationships for me.

Unbelievably, Mitch had the audacity to call me several months later as if nothing had happened. He must have spent enough time on the shrink's couch that he was back to his cocky self. He asked if he could come over.

Before I agreed, I asked him, "Should I invite Michelle, too?"

I never heard from him again.

# The Singles Bar

by
Sheila Moss

A number of years ago, I found myself suddenly single at mid-life. After recovering from shock, I began to realize that unless I intended to remain single forever, I had to seek opportunities to socialize with—yes—members of the opposite sex.

After mothering three children and living my entire adult life as one-half of a married couple, mustering up the courage to tackle the singles' scene was not easy. But I'll admit I was lonely. So I began to try to make the rounds of various singles' organizations and special-interest groups.

After figuring out that few available men venture into these women's places, I began to wonder just where all the eligible bachelors hung out. I spent as much time as possible at hardware stores—that seemed like a male place. And the advice books said I must attempt to create social opportunities while there. However, I could only lurk around the nuts, bolts and screws for so long before being suspected of shoplifting.

Finally, I came up with a bright idea. Guys go to bars to meet women. After I had tried everything else without success, curiosity won. I took the low road and decided it was time to hit the singles' bars.

By now, I had developed some poise in meeting people—not to mention my hardware expertise—and I felt confident I could handle most situations, including going to a bar.

Some women have shared with me that they have fun going to bars and meeting interesting men. I wish I could find those places. Whenever I go into a bar, I seem to magnetically attract the attention of every truck driver and wannabe songwriter in the joint. I don't know if they have radar or if I have "fresh meat" written all over me.

Once, before my eyes could even adjust to the dim light inside the bar, an Elvis look-alike approached me. "Wanna dance?" he asked.

*Well, I came to have fun, didn't I?* I thought. *He asked me to dance, not to get married. Why refuse and hurt someone's feelings?* So I agreed, and we stepped onto the dance floor.

All the decent-looking men were invariably busy with other women. Elvis, it seemed, came here often and knew the ropes. He glided too smoothly to the music and danced too close.

After the song, I excused myself and hid in the ladies' restroom for a while to regain my composure. Then I decided to venture out and look for a table in a dark corner where

Elvis couldn't find me. The trouble was that while I was losing Elvis, Bozo spotted me and started to move in.

"Can I buy you a drink, babe?"

*I'm not a "babe." But why argue? He wouldn't understand, anyhow.*

Bozo sat at my table without an invitation and told me the story of his life, including what a lousy bitch his third wife was. After five minutes, I realized why he had been divorced so many times. He was a loser.

Everyone smoked in the bar—it was hot and stifling. The music was too loud, the drinks too strong. *Is this what I have to do to meet someone?* I wondered. *Maybe I'd rather be lonely.* But I'd already paid the cover charge, so I stayed. I smiled, I danced and I listened to all the stories and heard about all the disappointments, the failures and the lost loves.

After a drink or two, Elvis began to look a lot more like Robert Redford. *Maybe this isn't such a bad place after all. Maybe I'm too particular, too critical. Maybe I could date one of these guys . . . if it weren't for the cologne.*

The smell of Old Spice was overwhelming and left me guessing that one could buy the stuff in gallon jugs. *If I could meet just one decent man with a scent from the men's section of a good department store instead of the special from down at the truck stop, I'd be his!*

All the stories and guys started to blend like a country song. I tried to sort them into categories that my mind could comprehend: jerks, losers and assholes. So many ruined lives, so many lost dreams, so many construction workers. I'd never met a construction worker until I became single. Now I was sure that at least half the male population in the bar had to have worked in the profession.

I also learned that night that the men who were half-way decent were usually married—but "separated"—at least for the night. Eventually, I realized that it was easy to meet someone at a bar, but difficult to meet the type of guy I wanted to meet.

Robert Redford wanted to take me out to breakfast. I knew what that meant. I excused myself to go to the ladies' room then exited out the bar's back door.

Robert would be disappointed that I didn't at least let him walk me to my car and give him my phone number. Who was I kidding? He was probably already hitting on someone else.

*Fresh air never smelled so good!*

# Who's Sleeping in My Bed?

by
Bobby Barbara Smith

"This is ridiculous!" my sister Judy exclaimed, looking at the wall clock then out the back window toward the garage. "It's almost two o'clock!"

Having married men who were into stock-car racing, she and I had spent many evenings together as the guys tinkered away in the detached garage, rebuilding motors and transmissions. We didn't mind, and the weekly races were fun. We'd sit on those bleachers with a blanket to protect us from the mud slung through the fence when the cars slid around the curves of the dirt track. Judy even participated in the powder-puff race, placing second behind her good friend. The roar of the engines and the serious competition were exhilarating.

But the evening had drifted into the early morning and, trying to stay awake, we had exhausted every topic we knew.

Judy's green eyes snapped as she took command. "We're going to bed! I'll make out the sofa bed for us. You take our room. That way, you won't have to move the boys." My young toddlers had fallen asleep hours earlier on a pallet bed in her bedroom.

Sis handed out orders like a drill sergeant, and I agreed, grateful for the bed. Upon entering her room, I pulled the pallet carefully to my side, clearing a path for my husband. My sleeping angels never stirred from their slumber, and I was dead to the world the minute my head hit the pillow. I vaguely remember hearing the shower running, but I slept until I heard a male voice cursing as he stumbled over the boys.

I rose up onto one elbow when I heard the cursing and knew immediately that the man—clad only in a towel—was not my husband. And he was headed for my side of the bed!

I said the first thing that popped into my head. "Um, kiddo, I think you have the wrong bed."

"Bobby?" my confused brother-in-law said, now clutching his towel tightly and trying to step backward over the boys.

Then the two of us heard a commotion from the living room. Judy and my husband had both just discovered their new bed partner. I heard her laughing then the sound of my husband slipping back into his jeans. "It would have been nice if they'd told us," the guys muttered to each other as they passed in the hallway.

Once we had our husbands in the proper beds, I had to know. "Did you get into bed?" I asked him.

"Heck, yes! It was dark in there, and I assumed the sofa was *our* bed!"

We started laughing as we realized what had happened. I knew my husband's nightly routine well enough to visualize what had taken place. Each night, he slips off his jeans, climbs into bed then turns and wraps his arm around me, just under my breast. Tonight, he had to know immediately that he was in the wrong bed when he slid his arm over my well-endowed sister. I giggled loudly and was thankful that he at least had on his tidy-whities.

We heard laughter from the living room as my sister and brother-in-law discussed the mishap. "If I hadn't tripped over the boys, I'd have dropped my towel and slid into bed!" my brother-in-law, who was still in shock, told Judy. This triggered more laughter from us. It took a while to settle down as we shushed each other, not wanting to wake the boys.

That was not the last late night we spent together, but it was, by far, the most memorable one. Now before heading out to the garage, the guys—both wearing devilish grins—ask us, "Which bed are we in tonight?"

# Out of This World Sex

by
Pamela Frost

After the divorce, I swore off men once and for all. But my hormones had other ideas. When even my dreams became solo performances, I knew I had to do something—and quick. Despite my friends' warnings, I dove headfirst into the Internet dating pool.

George seemed like an ordinary man. On the surface, he appeared to be just what I was looking for. But the first warning bell should have gone off loud and clear when he posted no photograph on the online dating site. I was trying to stop judging people based on how they looked, because too many pretty boys had broken my heart. Their God's-gift-to-women attitude was wearing thin with me. No more. I was done with them. So the fact George hadn't posted a photo was OK with me.

After a few online chats with George—and, in retrospect,

too few—George and I decided to meet at a local restaurant and bar. I liked the place. It felt comfortable; the lights were low, which was good for a divorced single mom the other side of 30. OK, maybe 40.

This date was my first post-divorce online hookup, and I was nervous. I tried on everything in my closet, and half the stuff didn't fit. My closet looked like a grenade had detonated. *How much weight had I gained?*

Finally, I settled on the classic little black dress. Cliché, I know, but the dress was understated and coupled with funky purple shoes; I felt it set the right tone. I wanted to impress George. And I really needed to get laid.

From what I'd learned about George so far, I thought our date could turn into something more. Most vital was his acceptance and even joy in discovering I had a son. He liked kids but didn't have any of his own. Online, he didn't go on about his last failed relationship like most guys. In a word, he was an apparent contender for my heart.

I learned some important rules for Internet dating that night. Always insist on a photograph. Sure, many guys post a photo of when they were 10 years younger and 50 pounds lighter, but at least I would have had some idea of who I was looking for.

I walked into the restaurant at a distinct disadvantage—he knew what I looked like. The bar was at the back of the restaurant, and as I sashayed down the aisle between the booths, I scanned the crowd, looking for someone who was looking for someone.

That's when a man stood and smiled. Even in the dim

light, I knew I'd made a big mistake. I thought about turning around and slipping out, but George had already seen me. I just couldn't leave anybody sitting in a bar all night, waiting for someone to show up. I'm not that kind of person. Besides, I had made a resolution that I would no longer judge people on how they looked.

As I drew closer, I argued with myself that it was OK to have limits. It's not a sin to be overweight; I was carrying 10 more pounds than I wanted. But George was obese. There, I said it. Yes, I'm a superficial bitch. I reminded myself to look beyond that, which wasn't easy since he filled my field of vision with his powder-blue polyester leisure suit. He had obviously outgrown it a few years and a few pounds ago. And his pants hovered at his ankles, revealing dirty track shoes.

I did my best to smile as I shook his outstretched doughy hand. My mind raced. *What do I do?* My friends told me it was good to establish limits, so George and I had agreed to a one-hour meeting before the date. But as I looked at the askew wig on his head, I became desperate to find a way to get out of the bar without causing a ruckus.

I feigned interest as we exchanged pleasantries. I looked around to see if someone I knew was in the bar. No such luck. I was on my own.

Trying to make the best of the situation, I said. "So, George, I hope you didn't have trouble finding the place."

"No, just plugged it into the old GPS," he said, pointing to his head.

*So that's what's under that bad wig. Don't stare. Don't stare.*

I ordered the house specialty—a Monster Margarita. I

knew I was going to need it. It seemed like the thing to do since he already had one in front of him.

"Do you live nearby?" he asked.

*Danger! He wants to know where you live.*

"The other side of town," I said, being purposely vague. Meanwhile, my brain was trying to figure out who I could call from the ladies' room to get me out of here.

We followed the standard bad-date protocol. We went from the weather to kids to jobs and when we started on travel stories, the conversation took a definite left turn.

I asked George, "You travel much?"

He smiled broadly. "Oh yes, all the time."

"What was your all-time most-favorite vacation spot?"

George opened up and I almost became lost in his fabulous stories of all the amazing wonders of the world he'd visited. But I was still having trouble with that damn wig. It moved, seemingly on its own. Maybe it was the margarita, but I'll never be sure. They did pour heavy in that bar.

Not one to mince words, I asked, "Wow, how can you afford to travel so much? You must have a good job and great vacation benefits."

"Travel is my job."

"So you're like a travel agent?"

He chuckled. "I suppose I am."

"Why is that funny?"

"More accurately, I've been sent here to observe and make a report."

George ordered more Monster Margaritas for us. They were going down too easy. I reminded myself to take occasional sips and thanked my lucky stars that we had a local Care Cab to take me home. My friends warned me that it was dangerous to get drunk around someone you didn't know, saying that my blind date could drag me somewhere and do unspeakable things to me. Who knew what Mr. Leisure Suit would be capable of? But my date did have the most incredible blue eyes, which caught me off-guard. *Really? Could I be falling for the Pillsbury Doughboy in blue polyester?*

Drinking more, I hung on his every word. The way George spoke of his transcendent experiences at the Sistine Chapel, Machu Picchu and the Egyptian pyramids was mesmerizing. *Maybe I can overlook his appearance, talk him into getting rid of the wig,* I tried to convince myself. Then I snapped back to reality. *Whoa, could I be that horny?*

When the third margarita arrived, I asked George, "So with all the exotic locations you've experienced, what the hell are you doing in Medina, Ohio?"

"I'm here to find a wife. Demographics indicate that this as an optimal area to meet women who are ideally suited to cope with change. I think that might be due to your weather here."

I was a little flabbergasted that he just put it out there so boldly, like this was a business meeting or something. *Looking for a wife!* I was hoping to be swept away by romance; he was just looking for a wife.

"You're already a proven breeder."

My eyes shot wide-open, and I sobered up instantly. *This guy had to be putting me on. Where's the hidden camera?*

On the off chance there was a hidden camera and handsome

Ashton Kutcher was punking me, I decide to play along.

"Proven breeder, huh? How many kids am I required to have?"

"There's no requirement, per se. It is vital to . . ." George paused then changed his course. "I would like to have many children."

"Whoa. How many?"

"Research indicates that you might be able to bear as many as eight without irreparable damage to your body."

*Eight kids with Mr. Polyester? No way.* "You never said you wanted eight kids on the dating site. What's up with that? Don't you think that's something you might have mentioned before we met?"

"In the past when I posted that information, it resulted in no dates. Time is running out. I need to find a partner. We are leaving at the end of the month, and I don't want to be the only male without a mate."

"Leaving? Who's 'we'?"

"My team. We've been here for five years, and now our tour of duty is up. We must return home."

"Home?" I looked deep into his eyes, and it made me feel all weird inside. *Something's not right. He's not joking. Where are the cameras?*

He put his hand on mine and said, "I usually would ease you into this, but I really am out of time. I would love it if you and your son would accompany me home. You'd still have time to arrange things and say your goodbyes. We can come back and visit. It'll be the most amazing adventure you could ever imagine."

"What are you talking about?"

"Your profile indicated that you are ready for adventures and you'd like to get married and have more kids someday, so here I am offering you that."

"Just like that," I said, snapping my fingers, "and we go off into the wild blue yonder and live happily ever after."

"Precisely! That's what I'm asking. You get it. I knew you were the right one. I just had a feeling."

This guy was starting to freak me out. He was definitely a bubble short of plumb, as indicated by the wig. "And what is this five-year mission stuff?"

"We were sent here to live among you. Learn from you. In our technically advanced civilization, something of our humanity was lost. Yes, we are humans, too. Gone from this planet many centuries ago."

My heart raced. This guy was a lunatic. He looked serious. I checked again for signs of a camera crew and Ashton. If I wasn't getting punked, this just had to be some new reality show. A horrible warning screamed in my head. *Oh, God! They're going to find half-eaten parts of me in a landfill!*

Just then, I caught a glimpse of my friend Jane. Relief washed over me. With my back to Mr. Spooky, I motioned her over. As she approached, I gave her, "The Look."

Stepping aside, I introduced George.

Jane swung into action after one glance at the Blue Doughboy. "Oh, my God! I've been trying to call you, Pam! Tina said you might be here! It's Fluffy—he's been hit by a car! You've got to come now! I'm so glad I found you!"

Taking both of George's clammy hands in mine, I said,

"I'm so sorry. I've got to run."

I didn't catch what he said as Jane and I rushed from the bar.

Once in the parking lot, I leaned against my car. The night air felt wonderful, and I could catch my breath. I told Jane the whole story while keeping an eye peeled for blue polyester, a film crew truck, Ashton Kutcher or a spaceship. And there was no need to rush to save Fluffy since there was no Fluffy.

Suddenly, there was a flash of light in the sky. I gasped and pointed.

Jane said, "It's just a shooting star."

"Really?" I said. "Maybe some men do come from Mars."

# CHAPTER ELEVEN

# Men: Having Their Say

Some testosterone-fueled testimonies . . .

# Mammal See, Mammal Do

by
Ernie Witham

We were at Flipper's place. Well, not the real Flipper, of course. He's long since gone on to his great reward, which, I figure, is because he was such a good dolphin with good karma. That meant he got to come back to this place and spend time rescuing young, bikini-clad beauties from the perils of the sea.

"Are you staring at that woman in the bikini?" my wife whispered.

"Huh? No. Of course not," I said, looking away from the amply endowed woman who was about to climb into a large pool full of excited dolphins.

We were at Mile Marker 59 in the Florida Keys, visiting the Dolphin Research Center (DRC). "Over half of our family was born at the Center," a young woman told us as we joined a guided tour of the watery digs, "while other family members either have come to us from different facilities or were collected long ago by previous management."

I was concerned that maybe she'd been at the Dolphin Center a bit too long, calling these big sea mammals "family," but all of the staff did that. It was part of the dolphin/human-encounter philosophy. Matter of fact, the DRC lets regular folks like us climb right into the pool to play with the dolphins.

"Excuse me, you can't go into the pool," the guide informed me.

"The blonde with the rose tattoo on her shoulder got in," I responded.

"I knew you were checking her out," my wife said.

Turns out that in order to "have an encounter," we had to pay extra and attend a three- to four-hour training session first. So my wife and I decided to pay the basic admission fee instead.

At that moment, we passed a smaller tank with three members of the dolphin pod who shall remain nameless because, well, I can't remember their names. And, I hate to admit this, but they all looked alike. That's when a strange thing happened. Upon seeing the antics in the tank, our guide became red-faced and stammered, "Oh my, I'm sorry. Perhaps we should leave them alone." She quickly tried to lead us away to another small pool.

My wife and I looked at each other then at the three nameless dolphins that seemed like they were frolicking like all the others. We noticed there was a bit more bumping and splashing, bumping and splashing, and then, churning and bumping and splashing, churning and bumping and splashing, and then the splashing turned to thrashing. It looked like the three of them were caught in a high-speed wash cycle.

"Dolphin sex," my wife said to me, quietly.

"Cool." I took a photo to show all my perverted friends back home. "You know, I hope our next hotel comes with a hot tub."

My wife winked at me and pinched my butt, which only seemed to make our guide more embarrassed. I tried to ease her discomfort. "Looks like you're gonna be an auntie, again," I said. "Congrats."

I learned later female dolphins purposely (porpoise-ly?) "do the deed" with all the male dolphins so that none of them know who the father is. That way, there is no jealousy between the guys, and no one kills the pup. Also, they all have to contribute child support. After a few flings, the female can retire to . . . well, the Florida Keys.

I didn't find this out from our guide because she quickly changed the subject away from sex and began telling us the history of the DRC. It was interesting stuff, but not nearly as interesting as the X-rated pool. As she was spieling, we snuck back to the small pool, which was now calm. I expected to see smoke wafting up from a couple of dolphin cigarettes, but there was nothing.

"I don't know about you," I said to my wife, "but I'm not sure I want to climb into the pool with any of these creatures. I'm wearing aftershave."

"Let's go to Bahia Honda then. It's supposed to be a great beach," my wife suggested.

Bahia Honda State Park is located right under the famous

Seven Mile Bridge and offers access to both the Atlantic Ocean and Florida Bay. The water is almost 90 degrees, the same as the ambient temperature. It's the kind of place where tension dissolves.

"Man, this feels just like a hot tub," I said, settling into the warm water.

"I know," my wife said, then leaned in close and whispered, "Hold this, will ya?" She handed me her bathing suit.

I did a quick glance around to see if anyone was near us then slipped out of my suit.

What a feeling! We were naked, in public, in the tropics, in water so clear you could see all the way to the bottom—both of our bottoms. We did not have a care in the world. We were living on the edge! The possibilities were endless!

We both noticed the kids about the same time—a pair of preteen boys, wading right toward us. Their timing wasn't the best. Here's a little hint you won't find in the guidebooks, but I'll share it with you now, so you can file it away for your next carefree trip. Bathing suits are a lot easier to take off while in the water than they are to put back on. Also, our struggles were hampered by the fact that we were now thrashing around bumping each other and laughing so hard we couldn't catch our breath.

The boys stopped before they got to us and quickly headed back to the beach. The way I figure it, they'd probably been to the Dolphin Research Center and learned all about the birds, bees and mammals.

"Tourist sex," one of them probably said.

"Yuck," the other one probably added.

# Get Famous, Get Laid

by
Ben Baker

Somebody please explain this to me. In the movies, some guy who looks like Quasimodo after a train wreck runs around doing this and that and being "sensitive." And women in the audience love it. They go on and on about how much they would love to meet a man like that. Apparently, the disfigurement does not make a difference, and, in some cases, is a bonus. Judging from what I've seen the ladies do, a guy who's a cross between Bigfoot and the Loch Ness Monster and who likes flowers could be bachelor of the year.

The *Phantom of the Opera* is another classic example. The Phantom looks like he took a home correspondence course in do-it-yourself plastic surgery and flunked it big time. The lady in the picture falls head-over-heels in love with the Phantom. Furthermore, women in the audience get all mushy over him, too.

Some time ago, there was a TV series called *Beauty and*

*the Beast.* The beast was a man that looked like he walked off Dr. Moreau's island. Again, he was incredibly "sensitive." I read an interview with the actor who played the beast, and he talked about getting more fan mail from the fairer sex than Tom Jones ever thought about. He even got more panties and bras than Tom Jones, who is known for having a virtual rain of ladies' underwear descend on him after a concert.

When the network canceled *Beauty and the Beast* the first time, women around the nation went ballistic, with many threatening to tear down the network with their bare hands. Wisely, the network restarted the show, but at the same time reduced the quality of it down to the point where viewers—even the ladies—began dropping off like flies on a pile of poison.

Even in the original *Beauty and the Beast* fairy tale, the lady falls in love with the beast. It just happens that he turns into a prince at the end, but I'm sure she'd have stayed with him even if he'd have stayed a hulking monster. I just don't get it. Maybe the women think he has a gigantic dick or something.

Why do women get so mushy over the guy on the screen when he looks like something I'd use for catfish bait? These same women would not give the same guy the time of day if they saw him on the street. Yeah, yeah, yeah, Ron Jeremy gets laid, but he's paid to do it and the gals doing him get more money than he does. Jeremy is basically a life-support system for a big penis.

Gentlemen, I draw your attention back to your high school days. Remember the class nerd, the one who was incredibly sensitive, which was one of the main reasons he was a nerd in the first place? I . . . uh . . . this nerd couldn't get a date if he'd won the lottery and had a big one. But he could star in any one of the above stories and women would kill themselves to go out with him.

Why? I don't know, but I wish I did. Get famous, get laid.

# From Sea to Sex

by
Joe Mobley

It is a known fact that sailors aboard all-male Navy ships get horny. While at sea, jokes about a guy looking at his hand and exclaiming, "You sexy thing!" were standard. Having a date with "Rosy Palm" and her five sisters was the norm. And "whipping the rat," "choking the chicken" or "flogging the donkey" weren't terms denoting animal cruelty, but rather Navy slang for acts of self-gratification.

Sitting on the aft deck of a ship at night, watching the full moon sparkle off the ocean, evoked thoughts of romance—but it was only a sad reminder to sailors that no one had seen a woman in two weeks. Thus, getting drunk and getting laid were the first two things most sailors wanted to participate in when their ship docked and liberty-call sounded over the loudspeakers.

In most foreign countries in the 1960s, back when I

served in the military, the three classes of people that spoke English were American sailors, bartenders and prostitutes. The ladies of the evening only needed to understand, "How much?" and only needed to say, "Five dollars" in English. Their hands and touches on a drunken sailor silently said everything else.

These working women mostly appeared later in the evenings, when sailors had already had a few too many libations. Not all women in bars were prostitutes, but one could easily tell the difference. The woman who walked among the men, placing her hands where men liked, was not a woman there for only the drinks and music.

When our ship, the *USS Rich*, pulled into port in a seaside Middle Eastern country—somewhere near Mozambique or Madagascar—our priority was to get off the ship. The crew would be on what was called a "port and starboard" rotation, meaning that half of the crew could go on liberty the first night and the other half the second.

"Are you 'going over' tonight?" my buddy Arthur asked. "Going over" was Navy slang for going on liberty.

"Damn right, I am," I quickly replied. "I want to see some color other than Navy gray."

Bars closest to the waterfront were the most popular. Those were the easiest to find for a sailor stepping into a new country. Then, once intoxicated, the sailor had less distance to travel back to the ship. Having liberty the second night was good because the guys on the first night had already found the best bars and shared their knowledge.

One recommended watering hole—where I was drinking and

bullshitting with my shipmates—was at full tilt when the working women appeared. After weeks of having seen only men, an erotic caress from one of the women made it hard for me not to ask, "How much?"

"Five dollars," she replied.

My whiskey goggles, along with the dim light, made her look desirable. Hell, all women looked good when you had been out to sea for a long time.

"Let's go," I quickly said.

Leading me out of the bar, we jaunted through a dark alley to a small hotel. She greeted the desk attendant with a few words in her native tongue. He spoke fluent English, telling me, "Ten bucks. Five dollars for the woman, five dollars for the room."

Paying him, the woman and I proceeded to a door, beside which stood a tall black man. *Not here for a threesome . . . he must be her bodyguard,* I thought.

If sober, I would have said goodbye to her and the $10 right then, but being young and intoxicated, I knew why I was there. The man outside the door, who never spoke a word, gave me a slight feeling of trepidation.

Entering the room—more of a cubicle with no ceiling, and walls that reached up only 12 inches higher than my head—I realized privacy was limited. The small space wasn't intended for overnight lodging, and it definitely was not the honeymoon suite.

The woman undressed then lay down on the tiny bed. She lit a cigarette. *Maybe a smoke before, or after, but not during sex?*

After she had snuffed out the cigarette, I got hard at work. No foreplay required. The local alcohol—more than likely a cousin of American moonshine—coupled with my testosterone whipped me along like a stagecoach driver drubbing pull horses in the Wild West days.

With my mission accomplished, we both hastily dressed. Exiting the cubicle, I noticed the tall black man was still outside the door. He never moved.

As she led me back to the bar, I began to sober up a little. The dark alley seemed more ominous on the way back than it had during the trip to the hotel.

Entering the bar, I spotted my drinking buddies and hoofed it over to the table.

"How was it?" Mike asked.

"Satisfying," I answered. "Now I'm going to get totally drunk."

Mike helped me stagger back to the ship after I accomplished my second task, and this time, there were no dark alleys to navigate.

That was no doubt the strangest sexual encounter of my life, the kind that made me wonder if flogging the donkey might not have been a more prudent decision. It would have been cheaper and safer—and there would have been no hideous hangover the next day.

# Dare to Bare

by
## Michael Brandt

Age is just a number. And age sometimes makes us do crazy things, like jotting down on your bucket list "running naked."

The idea of running clothes-free was intriguing and mystifying to me. John Updike once said, "Being naked approaches being revolutionary." With great trepidation—worrying if I still "had it" at age 72—I signed up for a 5K nude run at a nudist resort in the foothills of California.

The dress code was simple: running shoes, hat, sunglasses and lots of SPF 50. I heard that what happens at a nude run stays at a nude run—this would be my opportunity to strip off my burdens, fears, stress and inhibitions and let it all hang out and bounce around. I would run in the full Monty—yes, completely in the buff.

I was apprehensive about visiting a nudist resort for the

first time. Pulling into the resort, I was greeted by race or-
ganizers, who were wearing only shirts. They directed me
to the designated guest parking area. After checking in at
registration, my race number was written with a Sharpie pen
on my right upper arm, similar to the numbering system for
triathlons. I was relieved to find they wouldn't pin a standard
race bib to my bare chest.

Naked in broad daylight, and surrounded by over 200
people who were all waiting for the run to begin, was a great
cure for my self-consciousness. There was a mixture of seri-
ous runners, less serious runners and naturalists, all look-
ing for a unique experience. Everyone appeared to follow
unwritten etiquette protocols—personal space was respected
and no inappropriate comments, manual manipulations or
erections were noted. Most runners wore sunglasses, which
made me wonder if some had "wandering eye-tis."

Participants came in all sizes and shapes. Males domi-
nated the run and generally had similar packages, ranging
from diminutive penises to well-hung junk. Like most, I was
in the middle comfort zone, one that didn't freak anyone out
or draw undue attention. Unfortunately, men didn't have the
option of donning jock straps, which would have been dif-
ficult should a runner suffer from elephantitis. Thus, this left
me in only my running socks and shoes.

Females represented 10 percent of the field, and it was
evident that many just liked being nude and enjoyed tak-
ing their clothes off in front of 200 wide-eyed men. Well-
endowed females wore sports bras to avoid bodily injury or
self-inflicted pain. A handful had shaved their down-unders

completely or had a well-maintained strip, while others were nicely manicured or wildly carefree. For me, this was a hedonistic moment—one of pure self-indulgence. Can you blame me?

While in the assembly area, I noticed a female in her late 50s or early 60s staring intently in my direction. Her noticeable fixation caused awkwardness on my part; I searched my memory, wondering if we had had a relationship in the distant past. Or maybe she was gaping at my penis in wonderment? One thing that was evident—she was *not* ogling my running shoes!

I studied her face carefully through my darkened sunglasses, and then scanned her body discreetly, determining if it was familiar territory. Although disturbing, I soon realized she was staring at the 12-inch keloid scar on my chest from heart surgery four years earlier. It was a sigh of relief, but at the same time, disappointment.

At 9 A.M., the race started. It is the only race I have run where at the starting line, no one got close to anyone else. In most races—like the Boston or New York marathons—runners anxiously crowded the starting line, getting into a runner's pose, leaning forward with their right foot planted slightly behind them. They would set their GPS watches and take off like a dart when the gun sounded.

But when the gun went off for this race, all one could see was swinging elbows, bouncing testicles and breasts and butts in motion. No one dared to bend over in a starter running pose! The run had no time limit for the finish, which took the pressure off the slower walkers who wanted to work on their suntans.

I felt comfortable and surprisingly natural running through the foothills with my fellow runners, all in our birthday suits. Although this was not an endurance run, the course was challenging—a mix of asphalt, dirt fire roads and hiking trails, laced with scrub brush. At an elevation of several thousand feet, the panoramic views were spectacular. But my favorite views were of the ladies running in front of me!

At the end of the course, the sidelines were crowded with nudists forming a chute and cheering on the runners as they crossed the finish line. The sensation of running without clothes was surprisingly good. Running naked—like an ancient Greek Olympian—was so much fun, I wish I could do it often with the breeze blowing over all my skin . . . and especially my not-so-private parts areas.

I've run all over the world, from 5Ks to marathons, but had never run in an organized nude race. And I had never won an award for my age group. But I did receive an award at the nude run—third place medal for age 70+ male finishers. What amazed me was that both of these first-time achievements were sandwiched into one incredible day. At 72 years old, this crazy old man can still do it!

# Just Say Yes!

by
Timothy Martin

To paraphrase American female author Flannery O'Conner, "A good man is hard to find, especially a mature one."

Most men simply refuse to grow old gracefully. Instead, they desperately hide their true colors as they approach the autumn of their lives. Age seems to trigger nothing but anger and frustration in them. These same men, like Hugh Hefner and Donald Trump, often seek out younger consorts to salve their tired, bruised egos. How much younger? Well, let's just say that some of these women choose their breakfast cereal not for the taste, but for the toy.

Thankfully, the same cannot be said for mature women. The majority of them are like a fine bottle of wine; they mellow and improve with age. Older women, whose stock is thought to decline precipitously over the years, become more sensual and enlightened. After decades of being chained to kids and career pressures, they flower and come alive mentally, physically and spiritually. By the time they hit age 60, their feminine appeal exceeds anything you have ever witnessed. A mature woman can take your breath away.

There's a lot to love about older women. They know what they want, but they are smart enough to compromise when it counts. They've learned that life and love—including sex—isn't the way it lays out in most romance novels or movies, and that's OK with them. If they are in a relationship, it's usually because they want to be in one, not because they have to be. They know that healthy love is built on honesty and trust. Romance doesn't ebb off with age. When an older woman gets over the hill, she just picks up speed.

Senior ladies express gratitude for the things you do. Sometimes, younger gals take their relationships for granted, and that's a huge mistake. Men like to feel valued and appreciated, too, whether it's repairing a fan belt on her car, bringing her flowers or fixing her a romantic dinner. Young women often require a good deal of "financial gratification." Personally, I prefer to feel loved and appreciated for something other than my purchasing power. For that, it takes the company of a woman your own age.

Mature women don't do guilt well. Nor are they worried about broken dreams or unfulfilled goals. Age has deliciously mellowed them. They know how to feel good about themselves and their bodies. Over the years, women learn that an attractive person is one who loves herself, and that understanding comes from a place of wholeness and strength.

This mindset, in turn, attracts a much better partner, one not bothered by wrinkles or silver hair. It draws a guy who is looking for a woman of real beauty to grow old with.

It may come as a big surprise to some men, but sexual burnout is practically non-existent in older women. They grow more passionate, adventurous and confident with age. They are less prudish and inhibited in bed, too. Research reports that women between the ages of 60 and 89 who enjoy an active sex life have a better quality of life and are happier. They don't become lazy or weary when it comes to lovemaking. They see their partners as sources of pleasure. What's the reason for this? No pregnancy concerns, no phones ringing and no children banging at the door. With fewer interruptions, women can relax and enjoy themselves in the bedroom. Thankfully, those days of "sneaking a quickie" are gone.

Most men are aware that experience beats enthusiasm, hands down. For some guys, though, it's a tough lesson to learn. Particularly if they take their cue from men like Clint Eastwood, Hugh Hefner or Ted Nugent, who prefer to have relationships with girls young enough to be their granddaughters. What these men fail to understand is that love involves embracing your partner's body and mind. If a man 50 or older claims he can only feel affection for a teenage girl, let's call it what it is. Real men don't date children.

None of us are perfect in our relationships. We don't have all the answers. But the idea that men remain attractive as they age, while women do not, is just plain dumb, a cultural construction from a male-dominated society. Men need to take a much closer look at mature women and discover the true loveliness and grace that lies within each of them.

In other words, experience counts. Women get more confident in their abilities as they age and are more willing to go the extra mile. So do some men. As we grow older, we hopefully learn that sex is not just sex. It is a journey two people take together. Sex is both psychological and spiritual, and it makes us feel like who we are. As human beings, we identify closely with our sexuality, and it's an important part of our identities. We like to feel desired and desirable as we age. It's good for self-esteem.

A smart man will choose a mature woman over a truck-load of teenyboppers any day. You will too, if you know what's good for you!

# A Time of Renewal

by
Ernie Witham

Ah, spring, when a young guy's fancy turns to love.

"Let's stay right here in each other's arms forever," she whispered.

"That would be great, dear, except your parents are due home any minute now, and seeing us naked on their couch in broad daylight might be a bit of a shocker."

"Good point."

Ah, and a few springtimes later, when a middle-aged guy's fancy returns to love.

"Let's stay right here in each other's arms forever," she whispered.

"That would be great, dear, except the kids are due home from school any minute and seeing their parents naked on the kitchen counter in broad daylight might be a bit of a shocker."

"Good point."

And even a few more springtimes later when an older guy's . . . er, "advanced-middle-aged" guy's fancy returns yet again to love.

"Let's stay right here in each other's arms forever," she whispered.

"That would be great, dear, except we're baby-sitting the grandkids today, and seeing their grandparents naked on the office desk when they get here might be a bit of a shocker."

"Good point."

And now, here we are, springtime once again, when a guy who has no idea how the hell old he is finds himself . . .

"What in the world are you doing out here on the patio?" my wife asked.

"Ah, just pruning my bonsais."

"Why the heck are you naked?"

"I dunno, because it's spring?"

We both glanced at the patio table, and then my wife quickly said, "You might want to put on some clothes before Mario gets here."

Mario is a gardener, handyman and all-around good guy. He built my bonsai shelves, planted some Japanese maples for me, and put down our patio stones that weigh about a million pounds each. Now, I had yet another bonsai-related project to talk to him about.

I know, you're probably wondering why a guy with such "active" springtimes has now turned to gardening for enjoyment. Me, too. I mean, my only gardening goal when I was a kid was trying not to be around when my old man needed help planting or weeding or watering or picking.

"Where's Ernie? He's supposed to help me stake up the beans today."

"Said he had to go to school early."

"It's Saturday."

"Huh, wonder if he realized that."

I also had very little love of trees when I was younger, especially the kind that lost their leaves.

"Where's Ernie? He's supposed to rake the front yard today."

"Said he had choir practice."

"We don't even belong to a church."

"Huh, wonder if he realized that."

But life is full of roads less traveled, leading us to places we never imagined. Like me becoming a writer, for instance. I can't fathom bringing that up to my teenage friends back in my hometown.

"What're you guys gonna do when you graduate?"

"Work at the plant."

"Work at the plant."

"Work at the plant."

"Become a humor writer, exploring and expounding upon the lighthearted curiosities of everyday life."

"What?"

"Ah, work at the plant."

"Right."

For that matter, sometimes it's hard for me to comprehend that I traveled the complete width of the country and now live in beautiful Santa Barbara.

"Where're you guys gonna live when you graduate?"

"In a doublewide in my parents' backyard."
"In a doublewide in my parents' backyard."
"In a doublewide in my parents' backyard."
"In a condo in Southern California, where the morning doves sing while perched on aromatic bougainvillea plants."
"What?"
"Ah, in a doublewide in my parents' backyard."
"Right."
But time moves on. Besides, spring also means longer and warmer days. Too much direct sunlight is not good for my bonsais, so I was going to talk with Mario about maybe hanging some shade netting over my little trees to protect them.

My wife came back out onto the patio. "Mario can't make it. He's hung up on a gardening project across town."

"OK, guess I'll just prune for a while."

My wife cleaned off the patio table and put down a small bottle.

"What's that?"

"Sunscreen," she said, kicking one of her shoes over the patio wall.

"So nobody is coming over?" I asked.

"Nope," she whispered, sending the other shoe flying.

Ah, yes, I do fancy spring.

# CHAPTER TWELVE

# Shhh, Let It Happen . . .

. . . almost there.

# Fifty Shades of Play

by
Christine Cacciatore

Bondage. Spanking. Whips. Doms. Subs. Naughty, yet fascinating, words that generally have no place in my coffee-drinking, husband hand-holding, go-to-bed-early lifestyle.

Certain authors have glamorized the whole kinky sex thing and made millions in the process. With the advent of e-readers, there are no more incriminating book covers to hide. As such, no one knows what you're reading, making erotica available for the masses to enjoy.

It's everywhere. And I'm curious, because it appears spanking is not just a punishment anymore, but is also something people enjoy as a prelude to, or in place of, sex.

I approached my husband about it. I told him I was looking to write some erotica that contained spanking scenes. Would he be a willing participant in this experiment so I would know whereof I speak when I put pen to paper?

We've been married almost seven years, and I know him

well enough to recognize an interested gleam in his eye when I see one. If we hadn't been standing in the kitchen at 5:30 P.M. with our son sitting not 20 feet from us, his pants would have already been on the floor.

The agreed upon night arrived—at our age, we plan these things—and we were both giggling like naughty teenagers, swilling coffee to stay awake for the festivities. Right before bed, one quick shot of whiskey for courage. It would be painful, after all.

Before we set off for the sexual playground that was our bedroom, we set up the coffee maker for the next day and laid out work clothes. I tossed in a load of laundry. He brushed his teeth and skipped to the bedroom. I took my turn in the bathroom then joined him.

The lights were off. My husband lay face down on our bed, undressed except for a pair of red boxers with pink lips all over them.

I hopped into bed and gave him a playful smack on his rear.

He leaned up. "Did you put the dog in his room?"

"No talking," I ordered, with a much harder, less playful smack. I waited for a reaction. Nothing. "Feel anything?"

"Ouch," he said, laughing. "Not really."

I felt something, though. It felt as if I'd popped a blood vessel in my ring finger—it burned like fire.

"Maybe do it harder?" my partner said, sounding hopeful.

This was not going as I had envisioned. "I can't smack any harder. I think I broke a blood vessel in my poor finger. It's probably turning blue."

"Speaking of blue, did you take my blue pants to the cleaners?"

"No talking, slave!"

Forgetting my severely damaged hand for a moment, I delivered a palm-stinging blow. *Oh, the pain!* I turned on the bedroom light to examine my heinous injury. Sure enough, my ring finger had a broken blood vessel, and the entire digit was turning a lovely indigo color.

"Dammit. Yes, I took your stupid pants to the cleaners!" I was the only one in pain, and it was certainly not conducive to romance.

Turning onto his back, he yawned. "You probably have enough material now, right?"

*I do? After two swats?* It was at that moment I understood why a gag was sometimes necessary.

Giving up on erotica research for the night, I pulled my spa socks back on while he turned off the light. He then pulled me close until we were in our usual snug, vanilla nighttime position—warm tummies together, legs intertwined just so, arms across each other. We were both drowsy from the whiskey, despite all the coffee.

Right before I fell asleep, he gave me a slow, warm, bone-melting kiss, and I was reminded once again why I married him. "Let me know when you need to do more research. That was fun," he said. Seconds later, the sound of his even breathing filled the room.

People who fall asleep so quickly have a clear conscience. Maybe my husband didn't need a spanking after all.

# Getting Lucky

by
Sallie A. Rodman

I put my last quarter into the slot machine and pulled hard on the big brass handle. Bells rang and quarters tumbled down the chute. It was music to my ears. A cashier came over and paid me my $200 jackpot.

Feeling lucky, I headed for the roulette table. I found a spot, bought my chips and noticed the admiring glances of the men.

It was the 1970s and my husband, Paul, and I were on a couple's weekend getaway to Lake Tahoe. It was our first trip after the birth of our 8-pound bundle of joy, born six weeks earlier. My mom had graciously agreed to watch the baby and our other two preschoolers.

I was so excited to fit into my clothes again. I wore the fashion statement of the day—hot pants and black patent leather boots. I added a classy black jacket and fishnet stockings to complete my chic outfit. With my shiny blond Sassoon haircut, I looked sexy and ready to take on the club scene.

Paul and I have different gambling styles. He doesn't like the slots, and I don't understand craps, so we would usually split up for a while and check in with each other from time to time. I liked to walk around the casino, and when my intuition would strike, I'd pick a slot machine. When I tired of slots, I would wander over to the roulette tables. But not Paul—he always headed straight for the craps table and stayed put. He was lucky beyond words, so I called him "Mr. Lucky."

Well, Lady Luck wasn't on my side, so my money ran out at the roulette table in no time. I wandered around, watching the crowd and enjoying being noticed. Finally, broke and bored, I looked for my husband.

I found Paul amid a huge crowd that was screaming and yelling at the craps table. He was rolling the dice and winning big. I sidled up behind him, not wanting to break his concentration.

My husband rolled the dice with a heavy-handed fling and yelled, "Come on, baby needs a new pair of shoes!"

"Hi, Honey. How're you doing?" I whispered over his shoulder.

"Well, hi, Babe," he replied, turning around.

Immediately, the croupier stopped the game and in a stern tone said to Paul, "Sir, is she bothering you?" You could have heard a pin drop. All eyes were on us.

"No, she's my wife!" my husband said indignantly.

The croupier became flustered and asked to be replaced.

I nudged Paul. "What's going on?"

"Oh, he thinks you're a call girl, out to snag a high roller. He's embarrassed."

"You're kidding, right?" I said as my face turned a bright shade of red.

"Well, in that outfit, you do look hot. How about I cash in my chips and take you up to my room?"

Getting into the character of the moment, I replied, "I'm not sure you can afford me, sir."

"Why, madame, I do believe I can buy your services for the night. I've never slept with a call girl before," Paul said, opening his hand and smiling. He had a fist full of $100 chips.

A slow grin crept across my face.

"Come on, partner. Let's cash in those chips and mosey on upstairs," I bantered. And believe me, that night Mr. Lucky got his money's worth . . . and I loved being his hot hook-up!

# Randy Randy

by
Morgan Malone

At 21, I was slim, fit but not athletic, and certainly not a contortionist. Or so I believed until I met a bad boy from North Carolina. His name was Randy, and he was.

Reeling from the pain of an engagement that I had just ended, I encountered Randy at a local bar on New Year's Eve. He was the college roommate of an old friend of mine and had ventured into the frozen flatlands of northern New York for a holiday visit.

There was an immediate attraction, and one thing led to another, as it often did in those carefree days, long before anyone knew about STDs or AIDS. We ended up as lovers before the New Year rang in. Randy was inventive and energetic. In our friend's doublewide trailer that night, we did it on the couch, every chair in the living room and the kitchen counter before we collapsed, exhausted and satisfied. So satisfied.

What began as a one-night stand became for me a twice-monthly, three-day weekend in North Carolina. I was completing the last semester of my senior year in college, waiting for law school admissions and working on my senior honor's project. So the round-trip airline tickets from Rochester to Raleigh that Randy sent were welcome, as was the mindless sex that awaited me. From touchdown late Friday afternoon to the crack-of-dawn flight Monday morning, we spent almost the entire time having sex.

He was tall and well-muscled from his job of wrangling a TV camera at the local station. Randy's honey-blond hair and mischievous blue eyes were set off by the year-round tan he sported. He was as strong and unpredictable as the waves crashing into the Outer Banks. After the quiet and conservative lovemaking of my ex-fiancée and the few fumbled advances of assorted college boys, Randy's aggressive thoroughness often left me gasping and rubber-legged. There wasn't a surface, location or position which he would not use to cram as much sex as he could into our time together. I was having fun, exploring North Carolina with my new boyfriend, keeping it casual and carefree.

But I had no idea how strong our attraction was, how deep our need, until one night in April 1975.

We had ventured up to Chapel Hill in his ancient cream-colored VW Beetle. He had graduated from the university there, majoring in drinking and screwing. Randy wanted to show me the charming campus and best bars.

After a hike around campus stealing kisses in dark doorways, quiet library carrels and secluded garden benches, we ended up at a Mexican bar/restaurant nearby. Randy regaled me with stories of his misadventures in pursuit of his degree in communications while he plied me with frozen margaritas. Tequila made me crazy. I got that deep, dirty-girl laugh, my hands started roaming and my lips told him everything my eyes promised . . . and more. I was getting close to dragging him either into the ladies' room or behind the bar . . . or onto the tabletop! We had to leave before we got kicked out for inappropriate behavior that bordered on the illegal. Giggling and holding hands, we climbed into the VW for the trip back to Raleigh.

How the man could drive a stick shift and still have his hands roaming all over me is a mystery. How he could concentrate while I leaned into him, kissing and nipping his ear, neck and anything else I could reach was a miracle. It soon became obvious that we were not going to make it to Randy's apartment or even the city limits without satisfying the yearning that was fast becoming voracious hunger.

"That's it!" Randy yanked the wheel to the right, pulling off the road. I had no idea where we were, but we were in each other's arms as soon as he stopped the car. The engine was still running, our hot breath fogging the windows on the humid April evening. Fingers flew, buttons popped, kisses landed everywhere.

"Stop," I moaned. We broke apart. My shirt was undone, my jeans were unzipped, my hair was tangled and I was gasping for breath. I had managed to pull his T-shirt up over his broad chest and unbutton his pants. We stared at each other.

"Why?" He groaned as he started to reach for me again.

"We can't do it here. Let's just get home before I explode!"

He sat back, considering. Then he pulled down his shirt, opened his car door and got out. I thought he was pissed at me and was walking it off. But no. He rounded the front of the VW, the headlights illuminating him against the darkness that surrounded the car. He pulled the door on my side open with a growl.

"We're going to finish this here and now."

"How?" I sputtered.

Randy reached in and shoved my seat as far back as it would go. With what he had in mind, he made no effort to recline the seatback, perhaps because the car was so old, perhaps because he already knew what he wanted and how he wanted it. First one long leg then the other climbed into the space between the Beetle's dashboard and me. He knelt on the floor, facing me, my legs spread-eagled around him. I was speechless as he reached down and raised my left leg against his chest. He pulled my jeans and panties off my hips and up my right leg. Pushing my garments out of the way, he left them dangling in the vicinity of my left knee. Then my right leg was up and over his shoulder. My blouse was still unbuttoned and soon my bra was pushed off my breasts.

I was panting. But still clueless.

"Get my jeans down, honey. I can't reach that far."

His pants were still unbuttoned. I managed to get the zipper down far enough so that I could push the denim down his slim hips. Thank God Randy often went "commando." I soon freed him from his jeans. He was as hard as a rock. I looked up at his face, contorted with desire, not sure of what to do next.

His big strong hands reached under my bottom, raising me up off the seat. My knees were near his ears, my bare feet pushed against the windshield. My head hit the roof of the car as he lifted me up. We were eye to eye. I could not have looked away if my life depended on it. His hands were shaking, whether from the weight of my body or his need. Then he lowered me onto him. I was jack-knifed in the seat, desire dripping from my forehead to my knees. I pulled up, using my knees as leverage, my hands braced against my door and his seatback. Push and pull, I was filled with Randy, filled with lust and need and, slowly, satisfaction.

We had been so ferociously aroused that I thought it would be over in moments, and maybe it was. Time stood still as we moved together. The windows were steamed. We were alone in our own cramped, humid world. I could feel him everywhere, from the backs of my thighs resting on his chest to my butt grasped in his strong hands. It was sensory overload. Suddenly, the orgasm slammed into me. I had not even felt it building within. As I convulsed with pleasure, he joined me, holding himself rigid as quakes of passion grabbed him, too.

We were still. The only movement was our chests expanding as we gasped for breath in the steamy, sex-scented air.

Passion pumps you full of adrenaline. You are stronger, more elastic, immune to pain and discomfort. But when it is over, you realize that you are folded up like a lawn chair in the front seat of a car that has a smaller interior than a broom closet.

"I can't move," I gasped. "I can't breathe."

"I can't, either."

We stared at each other for a second. Then the laughter erupted. How ridiculous we looked! How insane we were! I laughed until I cried, convulsing in near hysteria until I could feel him harden inside me again. Once, twice, three times and we weren't laughing anymore. We were holding on through another orgasm.

As the waves receded, Randy groaned and said, "OK. Wait for it." I didn't know what he meant until he reached over and opened my door. He pulled my right leg off his shoulder until it dangled to the side, half in and half out of the car. Then he let himself fall out of the car onto the graveled surface.

So there we were . . . Randy stretched out in the dirt, his butt almost glowing in the moonlight, his jeans scrunched around his knees . . . I with one leg hanging out of the car, the other bent, my left foot still resting on the dash, my jeans and panties sagging from my knee. My shirt was in disarray; my breasts were pink and glistened from our exertions.

Randy pushed up to his knees, wiping his hands on his T-shirt as he pulled it down over his flat belly and shrunken manhood. He yanked his jeans up to his waist and rose to his feet. He got the zipper closed and the button fastened before he reached into the car to pull me out.

Disheveled and a bit disoriented, I stood while he righted my top and got me into my panties and jeans. Then he gathered me into his arms, kissing the top of my mass of messy hair.

"Well, I've never done that before."

"Me either."

Then, together, "Not going to try that again."

Laughing, we scrambled back into the car and headed home.

We only lasted another month. By my graduation in May, we were no longer lovers. I headed home for the summer then off to law school. Too far away and too busy for those weekend trysts, we drifted apart. But I had learned something invaluable from Randy. Sex could be fun. It could be silly. Sex could make you laugh.

I never made love in the front seat of a Volkswagen again. But I did laugh many more times in the midst of passion. Many, many more times.

# The French Way

by
Terri Elders

"Let's drop by Aunt Lily's before I take you home," Bob murmured, opening the passenger door of his aging Plymouth. "I'll stop and pick up some orange juice and vodka and mix us a screwdriver."

I smiled. It was our third date, and though we'd been buddies for months, I still didn't feel the surge of animal magnetism for him that I suspected he did for me. Age 17 and completing my first semester of community college, I thought myself sophisticated for dating a returned Korean War veteran six years my senior. But so far I'd fended off any suggestions that we might be heading toward something more serious than good-night necking. I knew Bob's Aunt Lily had taken a trip to visit relatives in Minnesota, leaving him the key so he could water her houseplants. I hesitated. If I accepted his invitation, would he expect more than what I was prepared to give?

In the 1950s, females—even college frosh—never admitted to anything beyond an occasional shy reference to second base. And even then, a proper coed would duck her head, blush and explain, "Well, he tried to get to second base, but I slapped his hand when he started to slip it under my sweater." We'd all nod and agree.

Some of the more daring of us even admitted to the occasional use of a tongue but only to our very best friends, the ones we could trust not to blab to our worst enemies. We all had plenty of both—friends and enemies—and knew exactly who they were.

Bob slid in behind the wheel. "What do you say? I'll whip up some scrambled eggs with cheese," he added, trying to make a more enticing offer.

I glanced at the Elgin watch I'd received six months before at my high school graduation. It was still several hours before my parents would begin to wonder where I'd been. They had grumbled a little when I started college and I told them I expected to stay out past midnight, but gradually the complaints had faded away. I'd brought home good grades midterm and had just been appointed editor of the school's weekly newspaper, the youngest editor they'd ever had. I had my own column, "The French Line," a play on my then maiden name of French and a nod to the movie of the same name, starring Jane Russell, which had been released the previous year. I'd thought myself pretty racy, since that 3-D movie had been ballyhooed as something that would "knock both your eyes out," an allusion to the double whammies that the buxom Miss Russell was noted for.

Bob turned to me, starting up the car. He was waiting.

"Oh, sure. Why not?" I finally said. "Those eggs sound good."

Screwdrivers were a popular beverage that year among girls of college age. We all thought of bourbon as an old-folks' drink—kind of smelly—and rum as vaguely foreign, but not exotic. It was something sailors drank with Coke. Vodka, on the other hand, was nearly tasteless, if drowned in enough sugary OJ. Guys soon learned that young girls didn't screw up their faces at the thought of a mild screwdriver.

In his aunt's tidy kitchen, my date proved a man of his word, donning one of Aunt Lily's gingham aprons and scrambling the eggs. He'd made sure I had a refill of my OJ and vodka, though, before he began to grate the cheddar cheese into the egg mixture. When he was finished, he filled two plates and brought them to the table.

I'd never heard of adding cheese to eggs. I knew Bob had spent some time in Paris on leave with the Army, so wondered aloud if that's where he'd learned to make eggs that way.

"Yep. I learned a lot of things in Paris. You betcha! Just ask." He winked. "There's still some eggs left."

I blushed and accepted a second helping. Delicious. And after the screwdrivers and eggs, Bob began to look a bit more delicious to me, as well.

We nestled for a while on Aunt Lily's loveseat, nuzzling and necking. In between kisses, Bob would riff on how much he appreciated all things French. French poodles. French toast. And, yes, French kisses.

I giggled because I'd previously confessed I'd grown tired in junior high of boys sidling up and asking if it were true that my name really was . . . wink, wink, nudge, nudge . . . "French." And did I?

Bob laughed. "Oh, I know you do." He kissed me some more then began to unbutton my blouse.

I found myself wondering how far this would go. I didn't wonder long.

"I'll take off this silly apron," Bob finally whispered, "if you'll let me take off those silly panties." He yanked at the apron strings and flung the garment to the floor.

I couldn't believe my ears. Neither could I believe my urge to accept that trade as fair and square. Who was this animal I'd suddenly become, fueled on eggs and OJ, this sultry beast who slitted her eyes and panted agreement? Jane Russell had nothing on me.

Then, just as Bob's fingers slipped under the waist of my black nylon briefs, he groaned and jerked away, bent his head toward the floor and threw up all over Aunt Lily's gingham apron.

We stared at each other in horror. He apologized, and we cleaned up the mess.

"Is that the French way of lovemaking?" I asked in an attempt to break the silence.

He laughed and hugged me. "I'm screwed. But not the way I'd wanted."

A few weeks later, on Valentine's Day, he proposed. I accepted. And on our honeymoon a few months later, we finally played the rest of that game that earlier had been called on account of, uhh, nasty weather.

We made a pact. We wouldn't give up our OJ and vodka. But we'd make love first and drink the screwdrivers after. And we'd always end those special evenings with scrambled eggs with cheese. The French way.

Nearly 60 years later, I know well who my friends and enemies are. I'm confident enough to confess to both, and even to strangers and random readers of *Not Your Mother's Book . . . On SEX* that, yes, I did French. And how! So go ahead and gossip all you want. As the French would say, *Ooh là là.*

# Victoria Victorious

by
Jean Salisbury Campbell

A wet nose awakened me around six in the morning, nudging its way under my hand at the edge of the bed. The snout belonged to Victoria, my visiting "granddog," who often spent the night while my daughter Katie was out of town.

When my husband, Doyle, and I turned in seven hours earlier, Victoria had nestled into her blanket on the floor by my side of the bed. We adored her and thought she was the smartest dog we'd ever known—she could even push the button on a water fountain at the park to quench her thirst after playing—but Doyle drew a firm line at sharing our king-size bed. I reached down and scratched her muzzle, the way she enjoyed, and then drifted back to sleep.

Later, a large paw tapped my hand. I tapped back. Her other paw united with the first. She now had her full head and both paws on the bed.

An unsanctioned relationship between a cocker spaniel and a Doberman pinscher had produced Victoria, who stood over 2 feet tall and weighed 50-plus pounds. With her lustrous, feathered black coat, trimmed in brown and accessorized by a white bib, she looked like a Gordon setter with a sharp Dobie face. Beautiful and clever, yes. Bedmate, no.

"I need my sleep, Vic," I whispered, while stroking her head and ears. She inched her upper body further into the bed. I then withheld petting in the hope she'd lie back down. A hind leg plopped itself onto the bed, joining her head and front paws. All that remained on the floor was her left hind leg—a yogi in the making, for sure.

"Lie down," I said. She moved further into the bed, enough to teeter on the edge. No part of her touched the floor by then. She always had me wrapped around her little toe, and I had no heart for pushing her away.

"OK." I kissed her head and lifted the covers. "Come on in." I moved toward the middle of the bed to accommodate her size. "But you have to get down before your grandfather wakes up." *And don't tell him I call him that*, I thought.

Victoria made herself as small as possible, her back to me, her legs curled and extended slightly over the edge. *This isn't so bad,* I decided. I knew she missed Katie and her own house and bed. I hated for her to be sad.

I drifted off again. She seized the moment to stretch her legs, pushing her feet into the mattress enough to slide her warm, furry self firmly against me. I moved closer to my husband. Once again, we seemed to settle in. For a minute.

Then Victoria arched her back enough to touch me, while her legs pushed forward into what could only be described as a horizontal downward-facing dog maneuver. I pushed back against her to prevent further erosion of my space. She pushed harder against me.

Victoria's body temperature warmed me to an uncomfortable degree. I wanted to throw the covers off, but when I tried, Doyle stirred in his sleep. His back was to me, so I couldn't tell if his eyes opened, but I didn't want to wake him before his usual 7 A.M. alarm. Hints of daylight were visible where the drapes came together, so I decided to gut it out until almost seven, when I would get up and take Victoria outside. Doyle would never know about our little hot-yoga session. Once again, I felt the pull of sleep.

A more powerful thrust from Victoria soon sent me directly against Doyle's back and Victoria's fur into my face and mouth. *Well, Namaste to you, Victoria*, I thought, before turning over and wrapping myself around Doyle's body. If *I'm going to be warm, better from him than the fur ball that was taking over the bed*. Victoria turned herself onto her belly in her version of the child's pose, then rubbed her muzzle and wet nose against my bare back.

My spooning pose awakened Doyle, who rose up in joyous celebration. "Well, well," he said, thinking he was about to get lucky. He turned his head toward me and came in for a kiss. At the same time, the unseen-by-Doyle Victoria raised her head to meet his. She rolled her tongue up the length of his face—chin to forehead—and then smiled.

I held my breath, unsure of how this ménage à trois

overture would be received. Doyle laughed and laughed and shook his head. I laughed even harder. Relief does that. Now practically in the middle of the bed, Victoria put her head on her paws and went to sleep.

# *Ay, Caramba!*

by
### Ryma Shohami

At five minutes to midnight, the handsome, seriously inebriated New Yorker meandered over to the festively decorated cement peninsula jutting out into the pool. Much to the consternation of his girlfriend, he began a slow striptease under the potted palm.

The other hotel guests, their scrumptious New Year's Eve meal now history, urged the exhibitionist on with catcalls and rhythmic clapping. His lewd gyrations synched perfectly with the beat of the mariachi band. Or did the musicians decide to get into the spirit of the evening and adjust their playing to his moves? Anything was possible on this balmy, romantic Puerto Vallarta night.

With each discarded garment, the audience became quieter; no one quite believed that he would strip all the way. After a couple of minutes, only a few titters disrupted the music. The children who had been allowed to ring in the New Year refused to be distracted by their panicking mothers.

At precisely midnight—just as the bandleader was flogging the swirling donkey piñata into an anti-climactic rupture, the brass instruments were blaring and all the waiters were shouting "Prospero año nuevo!"—the stripper cast off his Calvin Kleins and dove stark naked into the pool.

But now the party was over. The remains of the piñata hung forlornly by a thread, its goodies long ago grabbed up by the obviously untraumatized children who had witnessed the New Yorker's performance. This spontaneous entertainer, who had insisted on displaying his inadequacies in public, was probably asleep. Probably alone. And my best friend, Dee, and I were sitting poolside with that evening's dates, nursing a last drink and enjoying the afterglow of what had been the best New Year's celebration any of us could remember.

This vacation was a 30th birthday gift to Dee and me, a reassurance that the two of us were still young and sexy and that our respective divorces did not spell the ends of our lives. We had come to party. So far, Mexico had not disappointed.

Our arrival at the hotel had set the tone for the trip. Within five minutes of landing in the lobby, 20 hotel employees, from the lowly bellboys to the hotel manager, surrounded us. Fearing we had committed some cultural faux pas, we remained rooted as they all advanced.

By the time the fuss had abated and the desk staff remembered the other guests who had arrived on our shuttle, we were the recipients of enough party invitations to keep us dancing for a month. Some we threw away (we didn't come to Mexico to hang out with busboys); others we accepted (the manager had an American friend who had a friend whose uncle had a yacht). Ironically, our dates that evening, whom we had met on the beach, were from our home city.

We had almost finished our cocktails when I glimpsed someone at the far end of the pool area. He was young, adorable and even drunker than the evening's Chippendale wannabe. We watched with fascination his slow, weaving progress in our direction.

His path skimmed the edge of the pool, causing us to hold our breath as he attempted to negotiate all the obstacles. Then, as if in slow motion, he finally tumbled in, eliciting a collective gasp from our group. Before we could mount a rescue mission, his head popped up in the middle of the pool.

After bobbing around for a few moments, he continued his labored trek through the water, up the pool steps and across the courtyard, until he stood before me. With his long silky hair and large brown eyes, he looked like a dripping puppy. He spoke.

"You're so beautiful," he moaned.

"Thank you," I whispered, as much from surprise as for lack of anything clever to say.

My three companions could barely contain their laughter. The young man stared at me, seemingly speechless.

"I have to have you," he finally stated. Never underestimate the articulateness of a horny teenager. Dee choked on her drink. Any second, the hysteria would be unleashed.

"You can't have me," I sighed, with as much regret as I could muster so as not to crush his feelings.

"But why not?"

"How old are you?" I crooned, thinking to soothe his fragile ego.

"Nineteen."

"Well, I'm 30. I'm much too old for you." In those days, cougars were cats to be avoided.

"But I want you," he repeated.

Either this kid was made of tougher stuff than I had guessed, or it was time to discover what he'd been drinking and serve it to all my future dates.

Perhaps a different tack was in order. "Well, yes, I can see why you'd want me. I'm looking fantastic tonight. But trust me, in daylight my crow's feet are there for all to see." Actually, I looked about 23, and I had no crow's feet, but the goal was some gently delivered dissuasion.

"I don't care. You're so beautiful and I have to have you."

This was becoming tedious. Time to play nasty.

"Does your mother know you're still up and that you've been drinking?" I asked, sounding like a schoolmarm.

"I'm here with a friend," he slurred. "I'm going now, but I'll see you tomorrow at the pool. You'll change your mind." With that pronouncement, he staggered back the way he'd arrived, through the pool and into the lobby.

Two seconds of silence. And then uncontrollable laughter overtook us. Each time we thought we'd wound down, someone would chortle or snicker and send us all into another fit.

"So, you gonna take him up on it, or will you devastate

the poor kid?" my date chuckled.

"Are you normal? By tomorrow he won't remember this ever happened," I answered. "And if he does, he'll be too humiliated to show his face."

"I'm not so sure about that," chimed in Dee. "He seemed pretty smitten."

"He seemed pretty tanked. In any case, that's not my problem, is it?" I smiled sweetly.

"I think you should go for it," she drawled. "You know those 19-year-olds and their libidos. He's at his peak."

"I'm with her," my date stated.

"Make that unanimous," Dee's date piped up.

Their matter-of-fact tones belied the subject under discussion. They could have been advising me on a car purchase. I searched for signs of kidding, but seeing only sober faces, I decided that the evening had run its course.

"You are all perverts," I declared. "I'm off to bed. Sans the kiddie. Thank you for a lovely evening." With that, I gathered myself into what I hoped was a dignified stance, kissed my date goodnight and waved adios.

I was convinced that was the end of that. However, the next day, just as I had made myself comfortable at the pool, the hottie appeared and blocked the sun.

"Have you changed your mind?" he asked in all seriousness. My friend's soda spurted in every direction. I frowned.

"What's your name?" I asked.

"Del."

"Del, honey, what you're proposing is not going to happen in this lifetime," I lectured. "Please stop blocking my sun and go and find someone your own age."

"I don't want someone my own age. I want you."

I decided that ignoring him would be my best tactic. I closed my eyes and concentrated on the lively music of the pool band. He left with a promise to return. General MacArthur could not have been more dedicated to his mission.

"Do you believe that kid!" I exclaimed to Dee.

"What's your problem? A gorgeous hunk is panting after you and you're concerned with numbers on a calendar. You're on vacation! No one will ever know except for me, and I'm not telling. Live! Experience!"

Who had kidnapped my best friend and what had they done with her?

The next two days were a study in focused determination. Each time I climbed out of the pool, there was Del wrapping me up in a towel. Cocktails appeared as Dee and I lounged in the bar. And throughout all that was Dee urging me to, "Go for it!"

Was I nuts or was she?

On the third day, I was conceding that Del was funny and pretty smart for a 19-year-old. In the morning, I almost moaned at his sensuous touch when he slathered sunscreen on my back. After lunch, sitting opposite him while we played backgammon, I suddenly found myself fantasizing about the considerable bulge in his bathing suit. Glancing over at Dee, I caught a knowing look in her eyes and a grin on her face. Good grief, the two of them were starting to wear me down!

By mid-afternoon, I was generating more heat than the

wicked Mexican sun. Mumbling to myself that I would live to regret this, I looked around to see if anyone was within earshot, and fixed Del with a stern look.

"Room 1174. Be there in 10 minutes. If anyone is on the floor, you leave." I was about to screw a hunky teenager, but instead of enjoying the moment, I sounded as though I was conducting espionage. Was I really worried about a hit to my reputation with the hotel cleaning staff?

As casually as possible, I took my towel and headed for the lobby, sure that everyone knew what I was up to. Ten steps into my illicit adventure, I heard a high voice calling, "Del? Del, have you finished packing yet? We're leaving for the airport in an hour." Whipping around, I saw an attractive, mid-40s woman waving at Del.

"Not now, Mom! I said I'd meet you all at the desk," groaned Del, embarrassment and frustration oozing out of every pore.

Mom? Mom?! What was I thinking? Suddenly, the landscape rearranged itself and my potential afternoon delight was transformed into a cute, precocious boy who still traveled with his parents. Smiling regretfully, I waved goodbye and headed for the bar.

"Are you disappointed?" asked Dee as she slid onto the neighboring stool.

"Not sure," I mused. "It obviously wasn't in the stars. But I did learn something."

"Oh, yeah? What's that?" Dee asked.

"The next time a delicious 19-year-old insists I'm beautiful and that he'll die if he doesn't have me, I'll take his word for it. And I won't wait three frigging days to oblige, just to be sidelined by his mother!"

# NYMB Series Founders

Together, Dahlynn and Ken McKowen have 60-plus years of professional writing, editing, publication, marketing and public relations experience. Full-time authors and travel writers, the two have such a large body of freelance work that when they reached more than 2,000 articles, stories and photographs published, they stopped counting. And the McKowens are well-respected ghostwriters, having worked with CEOs and founders of some of the nation's biggest companies. They have even ghostwritten for a former U.S. president and a few California governors and elected officials.

From 1999 to 2009, Ken and Dahlynn were consultants and coauthors for *Chicken Soup for the Soul*, where they collaborated with series founders Jack Canfield and Mark Victor Hansen on several books such as *Chicken Soup for the Entrepreneur's Soul; Chicken Soup for the Soul in Menopause; Chicken Soup for the Fisherman's Soul;* and *Chicken Soup for the Soul: Celebrating Brothers and Sisters*. They also edited and ghost-created many more Chicken titles during their tenure, with Dahlynn reading more than 100,000 story submissions.

For highly acclaimed outdoor publisher Wilderness Press, the McKowens' books include *Best of Oregon and Washington's Mansions, Museums and More; The Wine-Oh! Guide to California's Sierra Foothills* and national award-winning *Best of California's Missions, Mansions and Museums.*

Under the Publishing Syndicate banner, the couple authored and published *Wine Wherever: In California's Mid-Coast & Inland Region*, and are actively researching wineries for *Wine Wherever: In California's Paso Robles Region*, the second book in the Wine Wherever series. They also released *Best of the California Coast* in November 2014; the book features 800 of the best destinations to visit along the Golden State's 1,100 miles of stunning coastline.

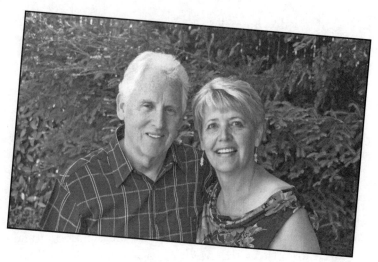

Ken and Dahlynn

# NYMB Co-Creator

## About Pamela Frost

If you were to meet Pamela Frost in a bar, she might tell you a stupid joke, like this one:

Q: How do you make a hormone?
A: Don't pay her.

That's not to say that Pamela Frost is a whore, but she did make you moan just now, didn't she?

Pamela's talents for sexual innuendo always make her the life of the party. If you see her in person, you might want to ask her what's so funny about peanuts.

Always the class clown, it was only natural that her writing took a left turn at funny, followed by dangerous "S" curves into sexy. Pamela said she got a little damp when she was offered another book deal by Publishing Syndicate to be the co-creator of *Not Your Mother's Book . . . On SEX*. All her life, she has wanted to say she wrote the book on *the* subject. OK, she edited the book on it, and it turned out to be almost as much of a climax.

Pamela co-created *Not Your Mother's Book . . . On Home Improvement*, where she worked with many authors who were publishing virgins. Her gentle editing skills eased them to a massive orgasmic release when their first stories were published in that title. The multi-published enjoyed the DIY partnership, too. She now relishes having done the same with those contributors in *On SEX*.

Pamela's debut novel *Houses of Cards* won an Independent Publishers Book Award in 2010. It's the story of a family who tried to get rich quick flipping houses and their hilarious misadventures. The book is available on Amazon Kindle and in paperback. She's also a contributing author in *Cup of Comfort for Mothers and Daughters* as well as many of the *Not Your Mother's Book* editions.

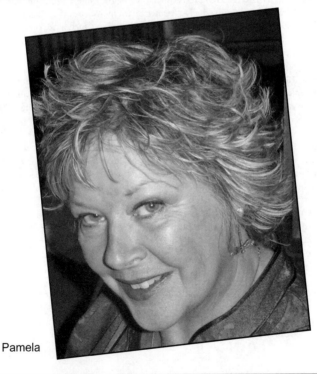

Pamela

# Contributor Bios

**Ben Baker** is covert ops in the world of humor writing. A pundit and syndicated humor columnist, he is also a professional curmudgeon. Ben's most recent books— *A Dog Named Nekkid* and *A Fisherman's/Liar's Dictionary*—were co-illustrated with his daughter Susan. Blog: http://porkbrainsandmilkgravy.blogspot.com

**Kathleene Baker** resides in Plano, Texas, with three adorable furkids—Hank, Samantha and Abby. She has been published in *Chicken Soup for the Soul,* various anthologies including NYMB, and in magazines. Kathy is co-creator of *Not Your Mothers Book . . . On Dogs* and the upcoming *Not Your Mothers Book . . . On Pets.*

**Cynthia Ballard Borris** is the author of *No More Bobs*, a quirky-misadventure. A humor columnist, she is a former board member of the National Society of Newspaper Columnists and frequent contributor to *Chicken Soup for the Soul, Not Your Mother's Book* and numerous publications. Email: cynthiaborris@gmail.com or visit cynthiaborris.blogspot.com.

**Michael Brandt** is an American author, international crime fiction writer and extreme adventurer. Michael has run over 100 marathons on the seven continents and has traveled to the four corners of the world. He lives with his wife in Northern California when not tramping the globe.

**Carol Commons-Brosowske** is a weekly columnist for *Frank Talk Magazine*. She has stories published in *Not Your Mother's Book, Chicken Soup for the Soul* and several journals. Her home and heart are in Texas, which she shares with her husband of 40 years. They have three children and one grandchild.

**Christine Cacciatore** co-authored *Baylyn, Bewitched* and *Cat, Charmed,* with sister Jennifer Starkman. Both are whimsical stories about witches with secrets (available on Amazon). She is married with three children and one granddaughter. She blogs at the "Life and Times of Poopwa Foley" and has multiple short stories published.

**Jean Salisbury Campbell** studied creative writing in Florida International University's MFA program. She has been published in *Chicken Soup for the Soul* and in a collection of fiction, *Everything is Broken, Too*, due on Amazon in Spring 2015 from Midtown Publishing. She lives with her husband in South Florida.

**Kathe Campbell** lives her dream on a Montana mountain. She is a prolific writer on Alzheimer's, and her stories are found on many ezines. Kathe is a contributing author to the *Chicken Soup for the Soul* and *Cup of Comfort* series, numerous anthologies, *RX for Writers*, magazines and medical journals.

**Sue Carloni** has been published in more than 70 magazines in the secular and religious markets for both children and adults. Among her credits are *Guideposts, Woman's World, Teaching Tolerance* and *Mature Living*. She lives in Wisconsin with her husband Kurt. They have two adult daughters and one granddaughter.

**Marlene Cloude** lives in Jackson, Missouri. Her writing career began when, unexpectedly, she was offered a position as feature writer for a weekly, total-market-coverage newspaper in Bedford County, Pennsylvania. She voluntarily produces and maintains five websites for organizations around the country. This is her first published short story.

**Darlene Cobb** is a retired school teacher/counselor who lives in Phoenix, Arizona. She self-published *The Dalmatian Without Any Spots*, a fictional story about a boy and his dogs. There is a very good moral to her story.

**Belinda Cohen** is a freelance writer in Pittsburgh, Pennsylvania. She's published articles in *Family Fun* magazine and *NYMB . . . On Working for a Living*. Her articles and book reviews have appeared on book covers and in many blogs, including everyfreechance.com.

**Shari Courter** and Ron have been married for 22 years. They have four children, a daughter-in-law, a son-in-law and one grandson. Shari has published stories in five NYMB books. She's a freelance writer, massage therapist and Zumba instructor. She also enjoys blogging her family's antics at closecourters.blogspot.com.

**Connie E. Curry** proclaims humor is the medicine of grand health. She is the author of *Katie Belle to the Rescue* and *Give Me Back My Glory*, a raw and humorous look at breast cancer. Curry, who resides in Delaware, Ohio, is the recipient of the James Thurber Annual Humor Contest award.

**Terri Elders**, LCSW, recently returned to her beloved Southern California. A lifelong writer and editor, her stories have appeared in nearly a hundred anthologies. She is the co-creator of *Not Your Mother's Book . . . On Travel* and the upcoming *NYMB . . . On Sharing Secrets* and *NYMB . . . My First Time*.

**Petey Fleischmann** retired from the federal government as a Purchase Card Cop (at least that's the affectionate term). She is enjoying retirement and lives in Woodland, Washington, with her wonderful husband, who goes out of his way to keep her on her toes.

**Karen Gaebelein** enjoys writing about everyday topics to engage her readers and make them laugh. Karen has won honorable mentions from the *Humor Press* and has enjoyed being published in anthologies. Contact Karen at gabe501@aol.com.

**Stacey Gustafson** is an author, humor columnist and blogger who has experienced the horrors of being trapped inside a pair of SPANX. Her book—*Are You Kidding Me? My Life with an Extremely Loud Family, Bathroom Calamities, and Crazy Relatives*—was just released. Website: StaceyGustafson.com, Twitter@RUKiddingStacey

**Julie Hatcher** is a freelance writer, wife and mother of two spirited young boys. She is currently working on a YA novel and other short stories. Her story, "Meow-thering," for the book *NYMB . . . On Cats,* is featured on www.LaughUntilYouPee.com.

**Stephen Hayes** is a Northwest humorist and creator of "The Chubby Chatterbox," a blog focused on humor, culture and travel. Hayes is an artist, traveler and world-class screw-up. His writing is an unabashedly sentimental exploration of growing up in the 1950s, 1960s and beyond.

**Renee Hughes** has stories in the *Not Your Mother's Book . . . On Dogs* and *On Being a Mom*. She's a CPA, has two grown children and lives with her hubby and rescued rabbit in St. Louis, Missouri. Besides writing, she enjoys acoustic guitar, church activities and alternative music. Website: www.squirrelb8.com

**Marion Hussey** began her career as a poet, but found that erotic writing was far more exciting. "Marion Hussey" is a pen name for a Los Angeles-based author who has been widely published in a number of national magazines, newspapers, books and on several websites.

**Georgia Mellie Justad's** humorous stories have appeared in *The Storyteller, ParentingPlus, Dew on the Kudzu, Midlife Boulevard* and *NYMB . . . On Being a Mom*. She's a transplanted Southern belle residing in South Florida, or what she fondly calls, "The Land of the Southern Impaired." Visit her at www.Justadshumor.com.

**Sherri Kuhn** lives in Northern California with her husband, daughter and a crazy yellow Lab. Her writing has been featured on *Mamalode, SheKnows, AllParenting, Huffington Post* and BlogHer, and her personal blog—"Old Tweener." Sherri was a cast member for the 2012 *Listen to Your Mother* show in San Francisco.

**Myron Kukla** is a Midwest freelance writer living in Holland, Michigan, the tulip capital of the world. He is the author of several books of humor including *Guide to Surviving Life* and two new e-books on Amazon.com—*Chomp* and *Something in the Blood*. Email: myronkukla@gmail.com

**Charlotta Ladoo** lives in Florida and is the queen of the one-track mind—sex, sex and more sex. This marks her first time published in an anthology; her story "Cyber Cherry" is excerpted from her upcoming novel by the same name. Website: www.charlottaladoo.com; blog: www.charlottaladoo.wordpress.com

**Rae Ellen Lee** is the author of humor, fiction and *neurotica*. Her award-winning memoir, *My Next Husband Will Be Normal* (available on Amazon), is a humorous relationship drama about a couple who moves to the Caribbean, where the husband soon realizes *he* is really a *she*. Learn more at www.raeellenlee.com.

**Juliette Lemieux** decided to "get her sexy on," offering a glimpse of her private life while most believe her to be straitlaced and reserved. "Juliette Lemieux" is a pen name for a Midwestern author who has published a novel, assorted poetry and stories in over two dozen anthologies.

**Morgan Malone** is the pen name of a retired judge and lawyer who now spends most of her time writing romance novels and memoir. She is the author of *Cocktales: A Dating Memoir* and *Katarina: Out of Control,* an erotic romance, both available in February 2015 from Turquoise Morning Press.

**Timothy Martin** lives in Fortuna, California. He is a columnist for the *Times-Standard* newspaper (Eureka, CA) and the author of *There's Nothing Funny About Running; Somewhere Down The Line; Why Run If No One Is Chasing You?*; and *Summer With Dad*. Email: tmartin@northcoast.com

**Siobhan McKinney** currently lives in Northern Ireland. She writes crime fiction and for a while served as an editor on *RAW* and *Paganman,* online men's magazines. Proud to claim the 2013 title "Poet of the Apocalypse" for a prize-winning zombie haiku, her four kids think Mom is a little crazy.

**Kelly Melang,** a self-made trophy wife, divides her time between Winston-Salem, North Carolina and Beech Mountain, North Carolina, writing for various local magazines. Follow her crazy adventures on her blog—"That Grey Area"—found at www.blueridgeandrv.blogspot.com. It is also available on Amazon and Kindle.

**Angela Miranda** is a veterinarian who writes because she can't shut up when something bothers her. Also, she's hoping for fame and fortune through writing, because she figures it must really be that simple. She plans to churn another set of autobiographical short stories into a collection titled *Autistic Stray Dogs*.

**Joe Mobley** grew up and resides in the riverside town of Swansboro, North Carolina. Some of his short stories have been published in *The Tideland News*, *Carolina Salt* and *Shoal*. His adventuresome youth and four years in the Navy set the background for many of his stories.

**Sheila Moss** writes a weekly newspaper humor column. She has been published in anthologies by Voyager Press, McGraw Hill, Oxford Press and in numerous other publications. She is past web editor for the National Society of Newspaper Columnists, founder of the Southern Humorists online discussion group and publisher of HumorColumnist.com.

**Amanda Mushro** is the writer behind the blog "Questionable Choices in Parenting." Sometimes she thinks she is doing a great job as a mom, but then she does something that makes her question her own parenting abilities. Her epic parenting fails and mishaps have been featured in four anthologies. Website: QuestionableChoicesInParenting.com

**Pat Nelson** co-created both *NYMB... On Being a Parent* and *On Working for a Living*. When not working on NYMB, she proofreads, edits, presents writing workshops, participates in writing groups and tries to learn more every day. Website: www.Storystorm.US.; email: Storystorm.US@comcast.net and Twitter: @PatNelsonWRITES

**Molly O'Connor** lives in Ontario, Canada in a century-old, three-generation farmhouse. She has published a collection of short stories (*Fourteen Cups*), a creative memoir (*Wandering Backward*) and a children's book (*Snow Business*). Her stories appear in four *Chicken Soup for the Soul* anthologies. She is now completing a fiction novel.

**Elaine Person**—writer, editor, instructor, speaker and performer—has had her work featured in many publications, including Random House's *A Century of College Humor*. She also writes under the clever pen name "Miss Elaine E. S. Person." Elaine invites you to visit www.Personalwrite.com for her "Person"alized poems and short stories.

**Cappy Hall Rearick** is a 2014 national award-winning syndicated columnist and author of six published books. A popular speaker, she teaches classes in Humor

Writing and Memoir. Read her columns, *Puttin' On The Gritz* at www.go60.us and *Simply Southern* at www.afterfifty.com. For stories and news go to www.simplysoutherncappy.com and www.simplycappy.blogspot.com.

**Sallie A. Rodman** is an award-winning author whose work has appeared in many anthologies and magazines. She received her certificate in professional writing from CSU, Long Beach.

**Candy Schock** has published more than 30 articles in such publications as *National Catholic Reporter, TWINS, Lutheran Women* and *Having Your Baby in Kansas City*. Her poetry has appeared in 50+ literary journals. She writes from the Land of Oz and can't wait until her daughter has to explain sex to her own daughter.

**Ryma Shohami,** a Canadian living in Israel for more than 30 years, is a technical writer/editor in the medical devices field. Her stories have appeared in *Chicken Soup, What I Learned from the Dog, The Ultimate Mother, The Ultimate Christmas, Wisdom of Our Mothers* and on Internet writing sites.

**Bobby Barbara Smith** is a writer and a musician/singer from Bull Shoals, Arkansas. Her humorous, heartfelt short stories have been published in several of the *Not Your Mother's Book* anthologies and in other anthologies and online publications. Bobby blogs at http://indy113.wordpress.com.
Website: www.BobbyBarbaraSmith.com

**Rosie Sorenson**'s work has appeared in the *Los Angeles Times,* the *Chicago Tribune*, the *San Francisco Chronicle* and other publications. She won Honorable Mention in the Erma Bombeck Writing Competition and is a regular contributor to the EBWW website. She also writes a humor column for the *Foolish Times*. Email: RosieSorenson29@yahoo.com

**Suzette Martinez Standring** is syndicated with GateHouse Media and is the award-winning author of *The Art of Column Writing* and Amazon bestseller *The Art of Opinion Writing*. Her work has appeared in *The Writer Magazine, The Boston Globe*, the *Huffington Post* and others. She speaks and teaches nationally. Website: www.readsuzette.com

**Laura Steidl** lives in rural Wisconsin with her horses, dog and husband. She considers herself a perpetual student of life and enjoys writing about personal experiences. Her story, *Benni Teaches Me to Trust in God*, is published in the book *Angel Horses: Divine Messengers of Hope*. (Allen & Linda Anderson).

**Jan Stephens** is the pen name for an author of a historical fiction, a book of poetry and several short stories. Although "Pink Roses" unveiled a side of Jan kept hidden too long, she is not quite ready to remove the veil completely, thus the pen name.

**Darcy Tarbell** lives in the San Francisco Bay Area. Her essays have appeared in such diverse publications as *356 Registry*, a magazine devoted to Porsche automobiles, as well as a journal devoted to Catholic thought, culture and action. She is employed in higher education.

**Ginger Truitt's** award-winning column has appeared weekly in Midwest newspapers since 2001. She has also been published in *Chicken Soup for the Soul*, church newsletters, her high school newspaper and, most notably, the May 1986 Barry Manilow fan club magazine. Follow her on Twitter (@GingerTruitt) or check out www.gingertruitt.com.

**Marilyn Underwood** lives in Fairway, Kansas with her husband, two sons and assorted pets. She writes novels and picture books for children and short stories and essays for adults.

**Stephen Vanek** lives in Dallas, Texas. He is a clinical social worker by day and a painter, poet and story writer by night.

**Phyllis G. Westover's** writing has appeared in magazines, newspapers and six anthologies. She received *Boulevard's* fiction award and was a finalist for the Iowa Award in literary nonfiction. Two documentary films she wrote aired on public television. Her children's book, *Sold to the Highest Bidder*, is available on Amazon and Kindle.

**Kathy Whirity**, a syndicated newspaper columnist, shares sentimental musings on family life. She is the author of *Life is a Kaleidoscope*, a compilation of some of her most popular columns. Kathy and her husband are discovering, with sweet surprise, that the honeymoon isn't over . . . it's only just begun. www.kathywhirity.com

**Marsha Wight Wise** lives in Baltimore, Maryland with her husband, three sons, four dogs and two cats. She is the author of four nonfiction books on local history (available on Amazon and Kindle). Marsha shares her day-to-day misadventures on her blog www.pulling-taffy.com.

**Ernie Witham** writes the nationally syndicated column *Ernie's World* for the *Montecito Journal* in Santa Barbara, California. He is also the author of two humor books and leads humor-writing workshops. Ernie is on the permanent faculty of the Santa Barbara Writer's Conference. Website: www.ErniesWorld.com

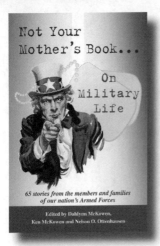
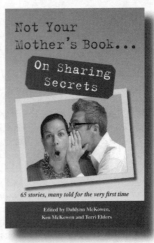
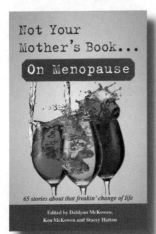
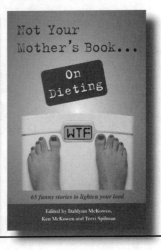

# Story Permissions

*Rockin' the Love Boat* © 2014 Kathleene S. Baker
*Get Famous, Get Laid* © 1997 Benjamin R. Baker II
*This Calls for a Thong* © 2003 Cynthia Ballard Borris
*Dare to Bare* © 2014 Michael Brandt
*Behind Closed Doors* © 2014 Carol A. Brosowske
*The Neighbors* © 2014 Carol A. Brosowske
*Fifty Shades of Play* © 2014 Christine Cacciatore
*The Special Blue Pill* © 2014 Christine Cacciatore
*Victoria Victorious* © 2014 Emily Jean Salisbury Campbell
*Doing It Where?* © 2014 Kathe Campbell
*The After-Sex Afghan* © 2014 Susan Carloni
*Games People Play* © 2014 Marlene J. Cloude
*Drugstore Jive* © 2014 Darlene F. Cobb
*Our First Time* © 2014 Belinda K. Cohen
*Slippery When Wet* © 2014 Shari Courter
*Wet Dreams* © 2007 Connie Evelyn Curry
*The French Way* © 2014 Teresa J. Elders
*Silence Is Golden* © 2014 Phyllis M. Fleischmann
*How to Buy a Plastic Penis* © 2014 Pamela Frost
*Out of this World Sex* © 2014 Pamela Frost
*Goofballitis* © 2014 Karen Gaebelein
*For A Good Time, Call* © 2014 Stacey Gustafson
*Whipped Cream Dreams* © 2014 Julie Hatcher
*Masterstrokes* © 2013 Stephen Hayes
*Peeping Toms* © 2013 Stephen Hayes
*Twice in One Day* © 2014 Renee Hughes
*My Visit to the Pleasure Chest* © 2013 Marion Hussey
*A Long and Winding Road* © 2014 Dierdre Jackson
*From Midget to Mammoth* © 2014 Samantha Johnson
*But It's My Birthday* © 2014 Georgia Melinda Justad
*Vaginaplasty* © 2014 Georgia Melinda Justad
*Booby Prize* © 2011 Sherri Kuhn
*Perfect Match* © 2013 Myron J. Kukla
*Cyber Cherry* © 2014 Charlotta Ladoo
*The Hired Man* © 2012 Rae Ellen Lee
*Coitus Calamitous* © 2014 Juliette Lemieux

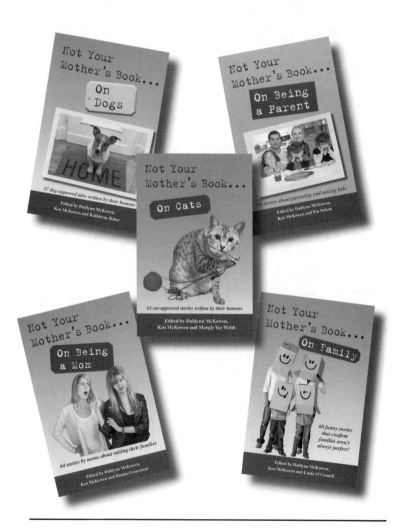

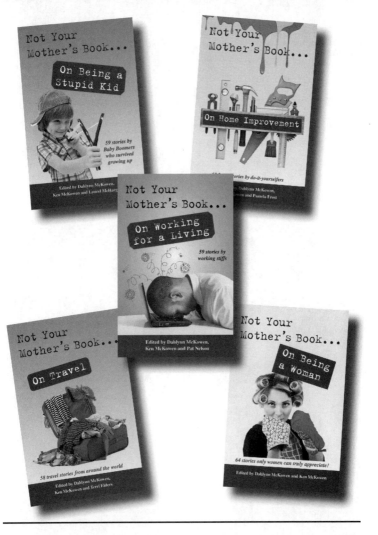